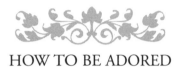

HOW TO BE ADORED

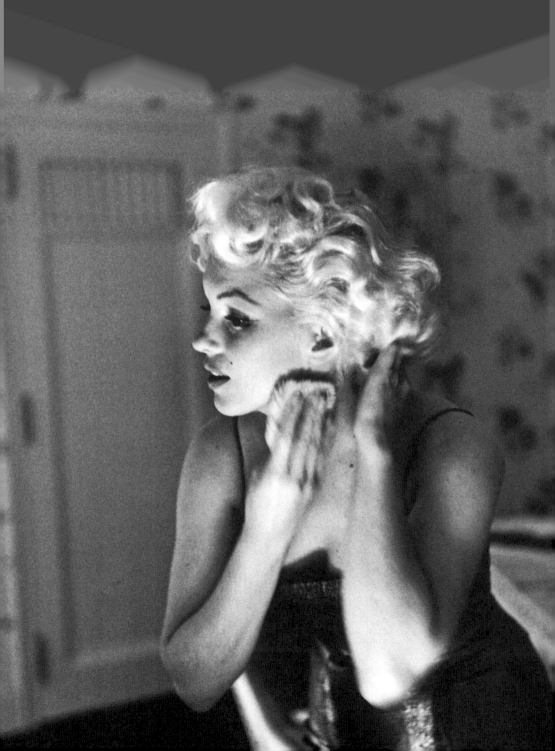

CAROLINE COX

how to be
ADORED

A GIRL'S GUIDE TO
HOLLYWOOD GLAMOUR

Quadrille
PUBLISHING

To Andrew, Joanna,
Lionel, Marnie and
Maggie — the most
adorable people I know.

Beauty, TO ME,
IS ABOUT BEING *comfortable*
IN YOUR OWN SKIN. THAT, OR
A *kick-ass* RED LIPSTICK.

Gwyneth Paltrow

This is a style guide with a difference. For the tips, hints, beauty and fashion advice come not from any old beauty guru but from a roll call of the world's most seductive women, including Marlene Dietrich, Marilyn Monroe, Audrey Hepburn, Brigitte Bardot, Debbie Harry, Jackie O, Kylie Minogue and Gwen Stefani. This book reveals their fashion and beauty secrets in their own words, but also those secret ingredients that make them utterly adorable – their warmth, charm and unique personalities.

Within these pages you will learn how to dress best for your shape, how to get Debbie Harry's smoky rock-chick eyes, Elizabeth Taylor's elegantly arched eyebrows and Marilyn's glossy red lips. But it's not all about the outside, adorability comes from the inside, so here you will learn to speak as eloquently as Grace Kelly, be as charming as Jackie O and have as many best buddies as Jennifer Aniston. Then at night when you lay your head on the pillow, like Drew Barrymore you can say to yourself: 'I was a decent person today'.

So crack open the Cava, open a box of Charbonnel et Walker truffles and indulge yourself with the ultimate guide to modern glamour: chock full of anecdotes, invaluable style advice and useful pointers straight from the lips of iconic stars. The world's most adorable women have advice that chimes perfectly for us now – because the lessons they teach us are timeless.

I
WHAT IS GLAMOUR?

WHAT IS GLAMOUR?

Marilyn Monroe was with friend Susan Strasberg in a New York street dressed down in casual clothes and wearing no make-up. Everyone ignored her until she whispered to Strasberg, 'Watch this.' Her body language changed, her hips swivelled – Marilyn had 'switched on' and the crowds suddenly clamoured for her autograph.

A true glamourpuss has just this brand of female sorcery, a form of fashion witchcraft that has the power to enchant and beguile. A woman of glamour has a magnetism few men can resist, *yet all of us can attain it* – even those without classically natural beauty. Many of the most beautiful women in the world lack glamour and conversely some of the most unusual looking women have glamour by the bucket load. This is because glamour is about artifice, as clearly displayed in the word's origins, *grammarye*, an ancient term for necromancy – the harnessing of supernatural forces.

The original belief was that magic had the power to elevate mundane reality – through the right combination of spells, the eye could be fooled into thinking that what it was seeing was something spectacular. In the early twentieth century, when glamour began to be used to describe a woman's physical presence, its derivation suggested that the artifice of make-up, hair design and all the frills and furbelows of fashion played the most significant part in making a woman look fabulous. Natural beauty couldn't always cut it!

GLAMOUR IS WHAT MAKES
A *man* ASK FOR YOUR
TELEPHONE NUMBER AND A
woman ASK FOR THE NAME
OF YOUR DRESSMAKER.

Lilly Daché
NEW YORK MILLINER, 1950s

My Glamour Secrets
by Marilyn Monroe

➤ Be yourself.

➤ Glamour is not all low-cut gowns and the slinky look. Blue jeans can still make you look attractive.

➤ Before you can convince others that you're attractive, you've got to believe it yourself.

➤ Enjoy the fact that you're a woman and men will enjoy it too.

➤ Trust your instincts – don't ask other women's advice on how to dress!

➤ Skim the fashion and fan magazines until you find someone who's your type. Then model your clothes on hers.

🌿 *The* Formula *for Glamour*

Is there a formula for glamour? Peter Noble and Yvonne Saxon interviewed many of the most famous female film stars of the 1950s and listed glamour's key ingredients, 'Take one part personality, add one part charm, another part sympathy and mix with a good complexion, a disciplined figure and a sunny disposition. Add a "clothes sense", personal cleanliness and daintiness – and the all-important quality of being able to make the best of yourself.' They added, 'You have no need to be a raving beauty. Your features need not be particularly regular; in fact, you can get away with a face which is definitely not pretty.'

And if you get the combination of these elements exactly right? Well, playwright Arthur Miller (who should know because he was married to Marilyn) thought it created a form of female power. As he put it, 'A beautiful woman can turn heads but real glamour has a deeper pull. Glamour has the power to rearrange people's emotions [and] to control one's environment.'

But, as this book will show you, with such heady power comes responsibility. For if you create the correct mix of personality plus an incredible dress sense to match your figure; if you conjure up a little bit of mystery and give yourself hidden depths; if you find your inner fabulousness, project it outward and become adored – you'll also have to spare the time to be warm, kind and charming. That's the difference between being admired like Madonna or loved like Kylie.

You Don't Have to be Born Beautiful

It should encourage us to know that while many stars and celebrities are born beautiful, just as many have made themselves that way or have been transformed by the stylists employed by the studio system (or 'star machine' as it was sometimes known in pre-war Hollywood) and the celebrity beauty industry today. In the '30s and '40s, studios such as Warner Brothers and Metro-Goldwyn-Mayer employed huge teams of experts to analyse each potential star's face and figure in minute detail. A report was then sent to the studio's boss, recommending the areas for improvement. On being given the go-ahead, specialist fashion, hair and make-up departments transformed quite ordinary women into gorgeous pouting ingénues.

Eleanor Powell's image is a perfect case in point. She was a wonderful mover – one of the greatest female tap dancers of all time – but considered a bit of a plain Jane by MGM. After the studio's rigorous physical assessment, its recommendations included:

- Grow hair from short bob to more sophisticated shoulder-length style.

- Use a special shampoo and hair extensions to give hair more volume.

- Perm hair into a softer, curled silhouette.

- Brighten hair with a rinse to make sure the overhead lights bounce off it during filming.

- Move hair parting from the side to the middle so as to draw attention away from a heavy jaw and re-emphasize good cheekbones.

- Reduce large pores with skin treatments.

- Pluck eyebrows into a more flattering shape.

- Use lipstick and lipliner to plump up a skinny lower lip.

- Grow nails longer and varnish them.

- Whiten teeth and cover any crooked ones with porcelain caps.

- Get rid of freckles with violet-ray treatments.

FOOTNOTE: Violet-ray was a popular therapy between 1915 and 1950. It used an electrically induced heat current that was passed over the body with a hand-held coil and was used to treat everything from backache to breast development (the equivalent today would be diathermy).

Extensive star makeovers continue at the same rate today with the help
of personal stylists such as Rachel Zoe (at least $6,000 per day), L'Wren
Scott and William Baker, who found the gold hot pants that re-ignited
Kylie's career in 2001 carelessly discarded at the back of her wardrobe
after she had worn them to a 'Tarts, Nerds and Tourists' fancy dress
party. The next day he coaxed her into them for her *Spinning Around*
video shoot and the rest, as they say, is history.

When Katharine Hepburn arrived in Hollywood, fresh from success on
the New York stage in the 1930s, the director George Cukor took one
look at her skeletal face and hooded eyelids cruelly exposed by hair
pulled back into a spinsterish bun and was appalled. He pulled her hair
free and allowed it to cascade to her shoulders, displaying its rich
auburn hue to full effect. He then ordered the studio hairdressers to
shorten it to chin length and concentrate on giving it lustre with a
series of egg shampoos. The new 'do' instantly showed off Katharine's
greatest asset – the most photogenic bone structure in cinema history.

Jennifer Aniston (reputed to spend $10,000 a month on beauty
treatments) has been transformed from a popular sitcom actress to a
Hollywood queen after a long layered haircut with golden tones that
cleverly drew attention away from a prominent chin and close-set eyes.
Her nose also seems to have become a little slimmer after an operation
'to correct a deviated septum'. And Angelina Jolie has moved from
being in her words, 'odd looking ... like a funny Muppet' – a Goth girl
with a solid black tint in her hair and a phial of her husband's blood
around her neck – to a woman of elegance and restraint in Oliver
People's shades and a wardrobe courtesy of American label St John.

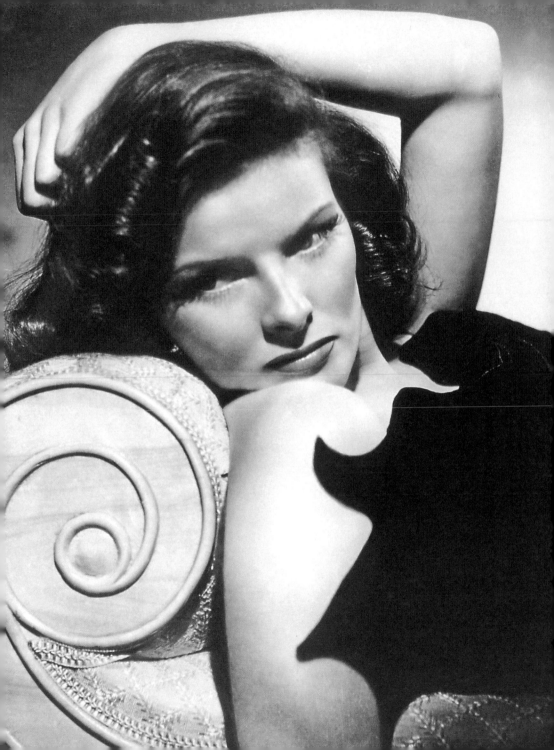

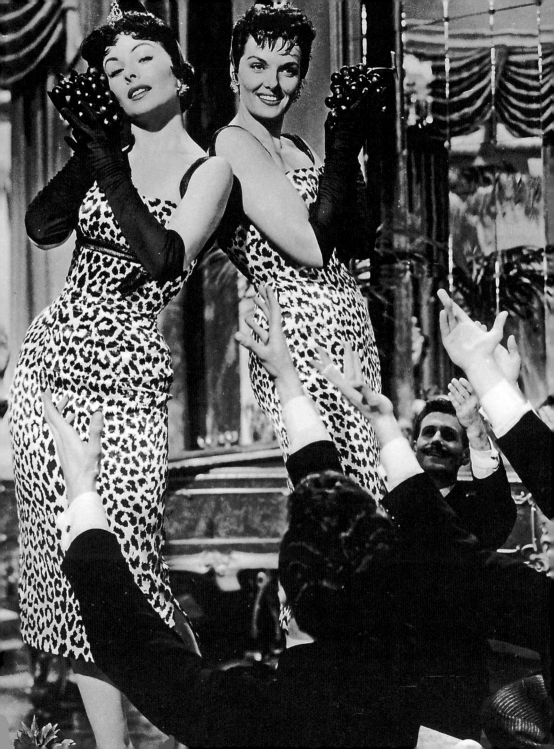

These examples took heaps of cash – but don't be down-hearted, the secret to glamour lies within reach of every woman. You just have to have the guts and the willpower to go for it. Put quite simply, you get out of it just as much as you put in, and true glamour will require some degree of commitment and hard work. Singer Gwen Stefani, one of the most breathtaking of contemporary stars, studies the glamourpusses of the past for inspiration and confesses,

'I'M *stupidly crazy* FOR OLD MOVIES. I RECORD THEM SO THAT WHEN I'M DOING MY MAKE-UP IN THE MORNING, I HAVE THEM ON. I CAN BE, LIKE, "*Look* AT JANE RUSSELL IN THAT *shiny leopard dress* – I'M COPYING THAT".'

Glamour is about creating a fantasy, and becoming truly adorable takes time. It's not an overnight transformation and you may find that at first it's the little touches of glamour that enter your life – a vase of white orchids in the bedroom, perhaps, or a little dab of Aqua di Parma Iris Nobile behind the ears as you hit the office. But you'll see, before you know it, it'll be seamed stockings every morning and an obsession with caramel-coated profiteroles! And as you emerge from your chrysalis as a colour co-ordinated butterfly, remember these wise words from '60s film star Arlene Dahl: 'There's no such thing as an ugly woman. *There are only those who have not realized their full potential.*'

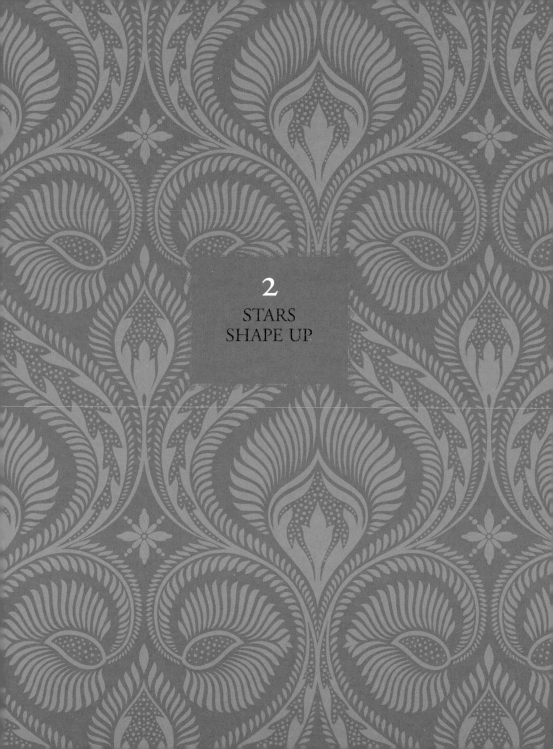

2

STARS
SHAPE UP

STARS SHAPE UP

Stars, like all of us, come in different shapes and sizes. Skinny may be in vogue today but the most successful icons of the past realised that vital statistics don't have to be that vital! It's a question of successfully dressing to suit your shape – whatever that shape may be. And here's your opportunity to find out as this chapter defines the key body shapes of some of the world's greatest glamourpusses. Compare your measurements with Ballerinas such as Audrey Hepburn and Gwyneth Paltrow or Hourglasses like Marilyn Monroe and Sophia Loren. Are you a Balcony like Elizabeth Hurley or a Pocket Rocket like Kylie Minogue? Or are you adorably Big … and Beautiful?

'A WOMAN'S *dress* SHOULD BE
LIKE A *barbed-wire* FENCE:
SERVING ITS PURPOSE WITHOUT
OBSTRUCTING THE *view*.'

Sophia Loren

✹ RIGHT: Audrey Hepburn's lithe proportions gave her a body meant
for fashion, but not designer shoes – she had size 10 feet!

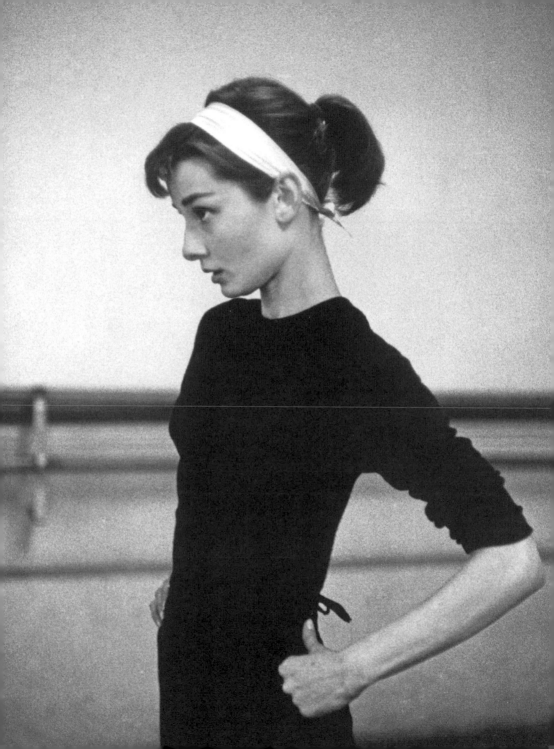

Ballerinas are lithe, lissom and elegant with a tiny waist and small bust. It's a figure type that goes in and out of fashion, at its height in the mid '60s with Swinging Supermodel Twiggy, whose celebrated measurements were 32–23–32, 5'6" (168cm), but a little dated by the 1970s when the glamazon bodies of Jerry Hall and Cheryl Tiegs reigned supreme. One of the most iconic Ballerinas, Audrey Hepburn was a refreshing anomaly in the 1950s, a Ballerina island in an ocean of Hourglasses.

AUDREY HEPBURN

In 1957 *Photoplay* magazine said of her, 'By any beauty parlour or beauty contest standard she is hopelessly ill-proportioned and unsymmetrical' – yet she went on to become one of fashion's most enduring icons. Today Gwyneth Paltrow, Nicole Kidman and Uma Thurman have the same bony frame and long swan-like neck.

Audrey stood 5'7" (1.7m) in her size US 10 (yes, 10!) feet and her lithe ballerina's body weighed 110lb. Her measurements of

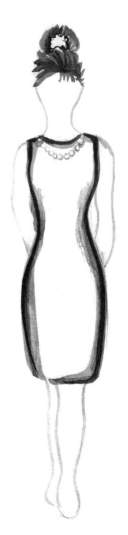

31.5–22–31.5 were maintained throughout her life by an iron will and determined self-control developed when as a child she endured the privations of Nazi-occupied Holland. Food had been so scarce that Audrey later recalled eating flour made from ground tulip bulbs and attempting to bake bread out of grass. As an adult she eschewed junk food and described her appetite as having 'a built-in leveller. As soon as I'm satisfied, a little hatch closes and I stop.'

NICOLE KIDMAN

In 2005 Chanel's design director Karl Lagerfeld was reputed to have described actress Kidman's body as 'bizarre... endless legs and not very much in the way of breasts. What she shows to the world is not her. Her perfection is an illusion: she knows it and couldn't give a damn.' Kidman is tall, standing at nearly 5'11" (1.8m) and her frame is notoriously skinny as a result of a combination of genes, yoga and cardio-vascular exercise – her dedication is such that she was spotted running with her trainer two months before the birth of her daughter Sunday Rose in 2008. Yet despite her enviable good looks, she's not entirely happy with her physique, describing it as 'a boy's body ... I would love to have boobs and a butt like Jennifer Lopez but I'm not having surgery to get it.' Like many Ballerinas, she towers over her partners – after her divorce from her miniature husband Tom Cruise 5'4" (1.6m) she announced, 'Now I can wear heels!'

If you are a Ballerina, you have a body made for fashion. Like Audrey and Nicole, you should emphasize your slenderness for dramatic effect – it's your best asset!

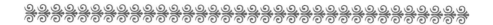

DO

➤ Wear a little black untrimmed sheath dress that will outline your figure, plus a string of pearls to show off your graceful neck as Audrey did in *Breakfast at Tiffany's* (1961). Her dress was by Givenchy but the sleeveless sheath is a classic shape that can be found on any high street.

➤ Buy full dirndl skirts and big bold belts to bring focus to your tiny waist.

➤ Use bateau necklines to hide your delicate collarbones – although this isn't a hard and fast rule. Gwyneth Paltrow, another Ballerina type famously wore a low cut, spaghetti strapped pale pink Ralph Lauren gown to accept her Oscar for *Shakespeare in Love* in 1999.

➤ Emphasize your body's naturally lithe lines with black and solid colours.

DON'T

➤ Buy outfits that don't fit correctly around the waist. A too short waistline will obscure your lissom proportions.

➤ Wear skirts that are too long. The Boho look won't work for you – you'll look like a child that has raided the dressing-up box. Audrey was ALWAYS elegant!

➤ Wear body-con Hervé Léger stretch bandage minis, and Roland Mouret Galaxy dresses are out too – you don't have the curves to fill them!

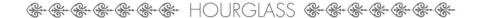

This buxom shape dominated the 1950s, a mammary-fixated era when women were at their most curvaceous. Jayne Mansfield, Marilyn Monroe, and Sophia Loren were all Hourglasses – a star shape that is defined by matching measurements for the bust and hips and a tiny waist in between – ideally 10 inches smaller! This sexy silhouette has almost completely disappeared from the modern celebrity scene, although happily we have Salma Hayek, Nigella Lawson and Scarlett Johansson to thank for keeping the Hourglass alive.

SOPHIA LOREN

Despite being nicknamed 'The Stick' when she was a child, Sophia Loren displayed one of cinema's most voluptuous figures in the '50s and '60s. She was tall for a female star – over 5'8" (1.75m) and with her stilettos and bouffant hair she could easily top 6 feet. This had its downside for male stars of the day – during the filming of *Boy on a Dolphin* in 1957 Loren had to walk in a trench alongside her co-star Alan Ladd so that audiences would be fooled into thinking he towered over her!

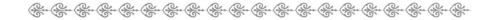

Sophia's measurements of 38–24–38 were almost too sexy. Lou Schreiber of 20th Century Fox refused to employ her, saying, 'Men are too frightened of her. She's too big, too powerful, too ballsy.' Yet Loren went on to win countless awards including an Oscar for Best Actress in 1962. She was well aware of her body's earthy power and revelled in it. When asked why she had stopped doing nude scenes, she replied with a smile, 'When Sophia Loren is naked, that is a whole lot of nakedness.'

MARILYN MONROE

Marilyn Monroe was definitely curvy – indeed, when compared with celebrities today she seems positively plump. She was a little shorter than Sophia Loren at a fraction over 5'5" (1.65m). Her hourglass curves fluctuated slightly throughout her career and measured between 35–37" (89–94cm) at the bust, 22–23½" (56–58cm) at the waist and 35–36" (89–91cm) at the hips. It has been difficult to verify her dress size as most were custom-made by the film studio so have no standard size labels. Whatever the case, she used clothes to emphasize and celebrate her shape. Marilyn seems deliciously curvy when viewed alongside modern celebrities. Fear of flesh is so rampant today that after seeing some of Marilyn's clothes in an exhibition Elizabeth Hurley said, 'I'd kill myself if I was that fat' and added, 'she was *very* big.'

How did Marilyn stay in such fabulous shape? Well, as she put it, 'I am a great believer in exercise, just to keep things in proportion. I am the lucky possessor of a small waist and some curves in the right places, but although I owe a lot to nature I also owe a great deal to careful exercise, plenty of fresh fruit and the right diet.'

DO

➤ Go for the full glamour effect – you know you want to! Think fifties burlesque – 'wiggle' dresses, stilettos, prom dresses and cascades of petticoats!

➤ Show off your chasm cleavage at all times with low cut necklines.

➤ Regularly wear a belt to cinch in that waist!

DON'T

➤ Wear all-over white – people will think you're a naughty nurse from the Fantasy Channel.

➤ Choose splashy all-over prints that many high street clothing stores think are suitable for the 'fuller-figured' woman. They are horrible and will make you look like a frumpy housewife on Valium.

➤ Obscure your delicious *embonpoint* with baggy, saggy tops.

➤ Wear minis, you will look tarty – a pencil skirt à la Marilyn will give you instant va-va voom.

Elsie Pierce's Guide to Feminine Loveliness (1930)

A healthy body is the foundation for beauty. Without it the eyes don't sparkle and the complexion remains unclear. Stars watch their health zealously in every era but some rules remain the same. Elsie Pierce, who regularly gave talks on 'feminine loveliness' in 1930s Hollywood, asked a number of shining stars the secrets of their twinkle and the results are very contemporary:

❧ Get plenty of fresh air – whatever the season.

❧ Do simple, general exercise to keep the entire system toned.

❧ Have a well-balanced diet, plenty of fruits, fresh vegetables, roughage – and not too many sweets, fatty foods and rich desserts.

❧ Water within and without – drink plenty of it – the body needs it – and take a warm, cleansing bath every night, followed by a cold or cool shower and brisk towel rub in the morning. The combination will cleanse and tone the skin.

❧ And DON'T. DON'T WORRY – for worry is the arch-enemy of beauty.

This slim-hipped and big-breasted look is today's fashionable ideal but a very rare body shape to come by naturally. It seems a little sad that such an artificial figure is today's most aspirational particularly when it requires painful surgery, or in Liz Hurley's case, vats of homemade watercress soup to get there. Stars who possess it (naturally or not – you decide!) include Angelina Jolie, glamour model Jordan and the celebrity formerly known as Posh Spice.

VICTORIA BECKHAM

This celebrity has taken an incredible amount of flack for her body shape, in particular in 2006 when a furore broke out when a spokesperson for David Bitton jeans revealed that she had a 23 inch (58cm) waist (the same size as Marilyn Monroe and an inch bigger than Audrey and Twiggy). Combined with her tiny hips though, this makes her very slim – especially after three children. Debates rage about Victoria's size and, on the face of it, her tiny frame raises all sorts of worries about why women are trying to disappear.

ELIZABETH HURLEY

Actress turned arm candy who came to public prominence on the arm of Hugh Grant in 1994 wearing THAT DRESS! Black, safety-pinned and very very low by Gianni Versace in 1994, it clung very snugly to her 36C–23–34 stats and catapulted her to celebrity stardom. After a long stint as the face of Estée Lauder, Hurley now devotes herself to her son Damian by billionaire Steve Bing, her Wiltshire farmhouse and her luxury beachwear range. It takes iron will and determination to get a body like this, allegedly one meal a day supplemented with a few handfuls of raisins for snacks – and a slice of self-obsession. As Liz says, 'I think I'm more concerned with body image than your average person who goes to work in an office all day. I do have to squeeze myself into a few dresses and bikinis. It's part of my job description not to be too fat.'

DOLLY PARTON

Country music icon Dolly Parton is artificiality incarnate and one of the world's most adorable stars. Her bust measurements are as exaggerated and enhanced as her hairdos – at a mere 5 feet (1.52m) she has a pair of boobs (or Weapons of Mass Distraction, as she dubs them) that measure a 40E and 36" (91cm) hips. Parton admits to having had her breasts 'jacked up a bit' and adds, 'My breasts have served me well – I don't know if I'm supporting them or they're supporting me! I was the first woman to burn my bra – it took the fire department four days to put it out.'

DO

➤ Be prepared for a lifetime of sacrifice.

➤ Wear bias-cut dresses to show off the fullness of your breasts and the slimness of your hips. Liz Hurley's trademark red carpet look is legendary. Gowns have to be designer (natch!) full-length, glitzy, décolleté and slashed to the thigh. As she puts it, 'I really concentrate on ways to look fabulous but covered.'

➤ Always wear sunglasses – the bigger, the better – they will help to draw attention away from your over-sized lollipop head.

➤ Take '50s movie star Cyd Charisse's example if you feel too skinny. Before dinner every night she drank a glass of sherry laced with a beaten egg.

DON'T

➤ Wear skinny jeans and flat shoes – with your bustline you won't be able to defy the forces of gravity.

➤ Wear Uggs, have platinum blonde hair extensions, use lipliner and carry a chihuahua – this is the working uniform of the Wannabe Wag and best avoided if you have any kind of IQ.

➤ Ever wear anything double-breasted – you're already double-breasted!

The pocket rocket is small yet perfectly formed. Lucky Pocket Rockets such as Kylie Minogue and Elizabeth Taylor in her prime have hourglass measurements on a miniature frame – others have less symmetrical proportions. Gloria Swanson, who seemed a towering superstar when descending a staircase as the psychotic Norma Desmond in *Sunset Boulevard* (1950) was a tiny 4'11" but dressed so flamboyantly she appeared 6 feet tall. Actress Natalie Portman at 5'3" is the same height as screen legend Vivien Leigh (who famously played the scheming minx Scarlett O'Hara in *Gone With The Wind*) but not her bust size. On describing her flat chest Portman relates a conversation she had with a costume designer, "'Right, this is where we push up your cleavage" and I'm like "What cleavage?"'

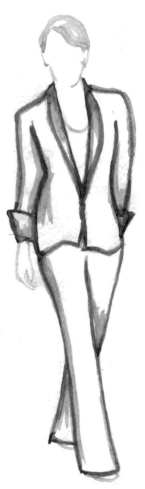

KYLIE MINOGUE

At just over 5 feet tall (1.5m) but a curvy 34C–23–34, Kylie has a little secret – her legs are disproportionately long on her small frame, at least 10 per cent longer than they should be – which is why she doesn't look overtly short. When further enhanced by her penchant for high heels and wedges, Kylie becomes the perfect Pocket Rocket and proves that tiny girls can overcome the 'Aaah ... isn't she sweet' tag and look as couture cool as the best of them. The pert symmetry of her bottom has been much lauded and had Justin Timberlake 'improvising' a rather raunchy grope at the Brit Awards in 2003.

CLARA BOW

Pocket Rocket Clara Bow gained international fame in the 1920s after being hailed as the 'It' girl by English novelist Elinor Glyn whose love story *Three Weeks* (1907), featuring a scene of 'sin on a tiger skin', had been a Hollywood hit. On being introduced to Bow in 1927, Glyn issued a proclamation in the pages of American *Cosmo* – 'Clara Bow has It!' When asked to define what exactly 'has It' was, Glyn waxed lyrical describing Bow's 'indefinable aura of animal magnetism'. At just over 5'3" (1.6m) the pleasingly plump Clara was a rowdy flapper girl who partied hard both on and off screen and cut a dash careering around Beverly Hills in her fire engine-red Kissel convertible with seven red chow dogs to match her flaming red hair. She was reputed to have worked her way systematically through the entire University of Southern California football team.

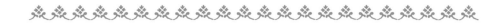

DO

➤ Wear V-necks, they make the body look longer – the same goes for block colour outfits.

➤ Always wear high heels – especially in bed!

➤ Wear fitted jackets to accentuate or create curves.

➤ Keep the silhouette smooth and slim. Bows and ruffles on those over 30 strays dangerously into Baby Jane territory.

➤ Keep accessories small and simple. You don't want your corsage to come into the room before you do.

➤ Choose hats with small proportions – a pillbox plus veil will give you a vampish air.

DON'T

➤ Wear anything infantile – dungarees, shorts, plaits and ra-ra skirts will have you carded at every bar, although your bus fares will be considerably cheaper.

➤ Wear any bold pattern in which the main motif is larger than your fist.

➤ Wear long skirts – they will make you look shorter.

➤ Wear a poncho – you will instantly become a comedy Mexican or a mushroom.

❋ RIGHT: A vision of art deco elegance, Clara Bow in 1931 shows Pocket Rockets how to dress like a vamp – you'd never know she was 5'3".

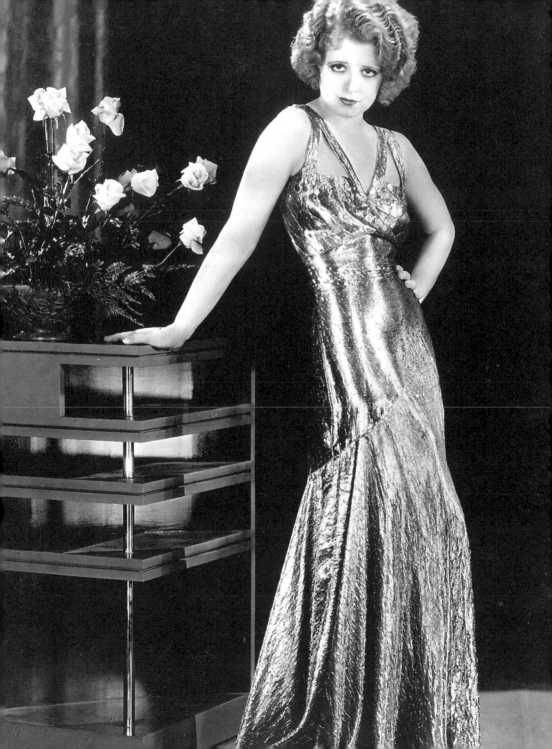

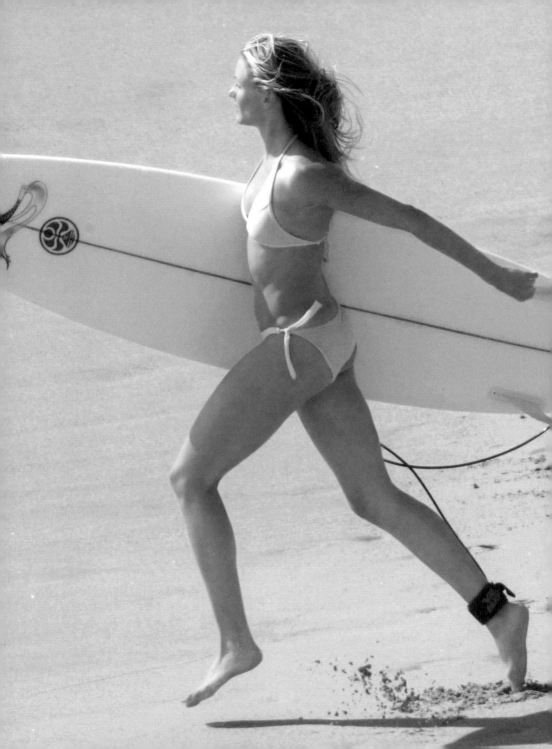

While some may see muscles on women as a violation of nature's laws, many find that attitude a little archaic today. The V-shape silhouette with broad shoulders and slim hips used to be considered entirely masculine but since the power-dressed 1980s it has become a new shape for any gym bunny willing to put in the effort. Athletes include Princess Diana, Cameron Diaz and Madonna. Many of the greatest glamourpusses had a similar body shape, in particular Greta Garbo and Katharine Hepburn, whose active lifestyles included sailing off Nantucket or taking in a round of golf.

KATHARINE HEPBURN

Hepburn seems to have hardly kept still – the ultimate tomboy, she played tennis, wrestled, rode horses and played golf. If she saw a hill or a tree, she climbed it and she could never resist ripping off her clothes and running naked into the pounding surf of the Pacific Ocean. She was nearly 5'6"(1.65m), slender rather than skinny and weighed 110lb.

✳ LEFT: Adorable modern glamour in the toned and athletic form of Cameron Diaz.

Hepburn's body was so androgynous that Greta Garbo (rumoured to have been one of her many female lovers) was supposed to have referred to it as 'the wedding of a man's body and a woman's'. Her great love Spencer Tracy was more succinct, 'there's not much meat on her, but what there is, is choice.' Author Zadie Smith, a lifelong fan, describes Hepburn as 'one long muscle devoid of bust but surprisingly shapely if seen from the back' and relates a story of the veteran actress crying with frustration at having a 24-year-old stunt double ride a bike for her in a film role – she was 72 at the time!

MADONNA

A practitioner of advanced Ashtanga yoga, Madonna is reckoned to have the body and constitution of an Olympic athlete. Her body fat levels have dropped so low that her biceps now bulge and her prominent rope-like veins are always clearly on display whether in a shearling gilet or the Versace dress she wore to the *Vanity Fair* Oscars party in 2006. She spent a cool £6 million buying the house next door to her London home to convert into a handy gym wherein her punishing daily workouts were said to include 400 sit-ups and the prodigious use of a Power Plate. As she puts it, 'I'm not going to be defined by my age. Why would any woman? I'm not going to slow down, get off this road, stay home and get fat. No way! I would never get fat!'

DO

➤ Wear clothes with slouch and ease, they suit your body's physicality – light tailoring is a must.

➤ Wear one-shouldered draped gowns à la grecque. Your toned shoulders and back are your best assets.

➤ Sport simple shapes in deluxe fabrics. Giorgio Armani's and Donna Karan's 'cashmere and diamonds' approach is perfect for you.

DON'T

➤ Wear anything too obviously sexy – toned doesn't go with tarty and with your triceps you'll end up resembling the local transvestite.

➤ Wear heels that are too high and attenuated – your calf muscles will stick out like a footballer's. You're meant to take elegant strides, not tiny baby steps.

➤ Ever go Goth – with your veins you'll be mistaken for a leftover lab experiment.

Our culture collectively shudders when confronted with Rubenesque curves, so much so that big, beautiful, glamorous stars are far and few between. Stars have become increasingly thinner over the years but there are a few sirens who have slipped through the net including the ubiquitous Mae West.

MAE WEST

Nobody is entirely sure of Mae West's measurements because even Edith Head, Hollywood's foremost costume designer in the interwar years, never saw her body out of a corset. Mae's physical presence was show-stopping; form-fitting bejewelled gowns struggled to contain her voluptuous body and showed off a cleavage that actor Anthony Quinn described as 'dizzying'. Her pneumatic qualities were so renowned that the British Air Force nicknamed their life jackets after her. If it could be so now! Singer Charlotte Church recently summed up the prevailing attitude to her own buxom charms, 'When I try to get work in the US all they say is that I need to lose weight – but I bet they never said that to Mae West.'

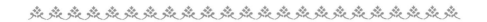

DO

⇥ Go tight, why not? When Mae West first came to Hollywood she told every costume designer, 'I like 'em tight, girls.'

⇥ Work with the impact of your physical presence. One Hollywood critic described Mae's entrance in a movie as 'a terrific explosion. A bomb had gone off in a cream-puff factory. Blonde, buxom, rowdy Mae – slithering across the screen in a spangled, sausage-skin gown.'

⇥ Slouch languorously with one hand on your hip. It worked for Mae, it'll work for you.

⇥ Look on the high street for clothes, they are there. New Look go up to size 26 and H&M has a well-designed B.I.B. range in UK sizes 16–30.

DON'T

⇥ Think you can only buy high street. There are some fabulous deluxe labels for the Big and Beautiful. Look for Ischiko, Oska and Shirin Guild, who design quirky high-end clothes that are designed for curves.

⇥ Always go by the standard label. Certain shapes can go bigger – Vivienne Westwood's jersey draped wrapped dresses are renowned among fashionistas for being able to accommodate some of the largest sizes!

Everything You See
I Owe to Pasta!
by Sophia Loren

'Women are obsessed by extra weight and many of them have made their lives very difficult by starving themselves into nervous weak creatures who are chronically depressed because they believe themselves to be a few pounds overweight. I have seen women at dinner parties who are so thin that their shoulders could be weapons and they eat nothing because they are "watching the calories". I have known women who have wasted years of their lives by believing they are too fat to be glamorous. They dread shopping for clothes, they hate to dress up for an occasion, they complain about the smallest bulge on the waistline or thigh as if it were a failure of the greatest magnitude. In Italy we call these women *attaccapanni*, which means "coat-hanger", because that is what they resemble.'

❋ RIGHT: Sophia Loren combines an earthy Mediterranean sexuality with an uptown feel for fashion and is a renowned cook specializing in her native Italian cuisine.

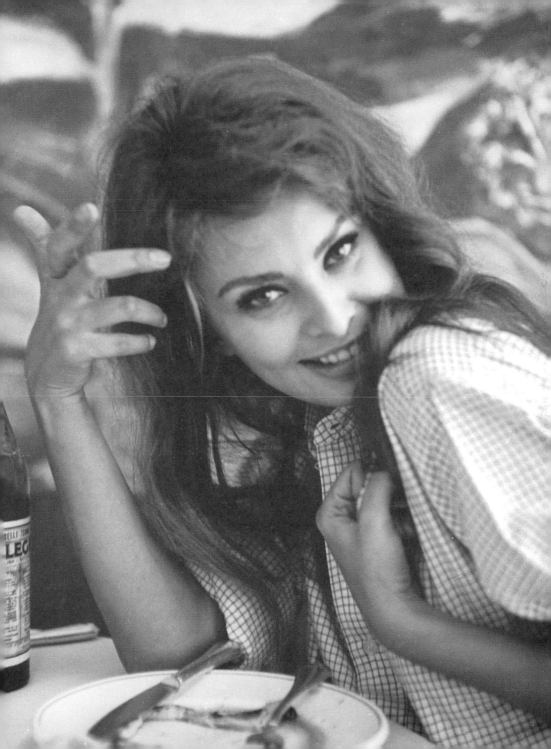

Celebrity Diets Revealed
... and Dismissed!

Fad diets appear and disappear as often as reality TV stars. They both enjoy wild success for a season then are put back on the shelf never to be heard from again. There's the Cabbage Soup Diet of the 1980s, which had obvious gas powered side effects, the early 2000s Atkins low carb approach once favoured by Renée Zellweger and Sarah Jessica Parker, and the Zone, a 1990s favourite that has recently regained its popularity with Jennifer Aniston and Cindy Crawford following its rules of different ratios of food eaten in measured amounts to regulate the body's production of insulin.

Whatever the method in favour, it's clear that the consumption of food has become something of an issue. Every age has its taboos – the Victorians were a little queasy when it came to talking about sex, yet they relished mealtimes and approached all manner of foodstuffs with gusto. We can face the most extreme of sexual practices with nary a hair turned but when it comes to confrontation with a cream bun all hell breaks loose. How do glamourpusses cope? Here's a selection of tips to muse on until you catch the eye of the maître d' at the Taste of Nawab.

EAT LIKE THE STARS!

ANGELINA JOLIE follows the Upside-Down Diet. Eat a gigantic breakfast, a tiny lunch and a minuscule dinner washed down with two litres of ice cold water to speed up your metabolism.

REESE WITHERSPOON is said to snack on babyfood!

SOPHIA LOREN 'Eat more pasta! I urge pasta upon you. How many times have people, while covertly gazing at my hips or waistline, asked how I keep my figure with all that pasta. Now the tag-along scientists have confirmed what Italian mamas have known for generations – pasta is good for you.'

MIRIAM HOPKINS banned fried foods – spices and tart sauces – and she stuck to three pet don'ts: Don't overeat, oversleep or oversit.

MADONNA eats macrobiotically. As she puts it, 'Fish, grains, some kind of grains. Some kind of cooked vegetable. Salad. Simple but tasty.' No meat, eggs, cream, cheese, salt, preservatives or sugar, and always organic. Chew 50 times per mouthful.

CATHERINE ZETA-JONES doesn't eat carbs after five o'clock and hasn't 'eaten chips since [she] was 14'.

CHARLIZE THERON says, 'Barbecue is a big part of my life. For breakfast, steak and eggs. But I will not mix sugar and salt like the American breakfast of pancakes, eggs and bacon. That's gross.'

AUDREY HEPBURN revealed,

'I DON'T LIKE *fancy* FOOD AT ALL. I MUCH PREFER AN EXTREMELY *simple* MEAL THAT'S *exquisitely* DONE ... A *perfectly* COOKED STEAK, A *beautiful* SALAD, SOME RASPBERRIES.'

ELIZABETH TAYLOR advises, 'Be a milk drinker. Milk is my recipe for a lovely skin, sparkling eyes and a well-rounded figure. Without any of these three attributes you cannot be called "attractive".'

BEYONCÉ KNOWLES goes on the Maple Syrup Diet if she has to shed pounds quickly for a film role, using Madal Bal Natural Tree Syrup. She mixes it with water, lemon juice and cayenne pepper and then drinks it instead of dinner for 14 days. After the filming she devours 'waffles, fried chicken, cheeseburgers, french fries, everything I can find!'

SHILPA SHETTY, legendary Bollywood glamourpuss, has a weakness for Godiva chocolates, custard and toast with lashings of butter. 'I wear a silver chain around my waist that rides up when I've put on weight. That's when I know I've gone overboard with my favourite puddings. The key to a good body is simple – eat well and exercise. If you are working like a dog and eating like a pig, it won't work.'

TYRA BANKS eats fresh fruit, especially mango, papaya and chicken and shrimp salad. She also has a part-time chef who is responsible for the evenings. 'He makes meals and leaves them for when I get home,' she says.

TWIGGY:

'I don't SIT AROUND *stuffing* MYSELF WITH *cream cakes.'*

Magic Word Diet
by Paige Thomas (1957)

'Our research has unearthed the one and only successful magic formula diet in the world. It is called the Three Little Words diet. You just say the magic words and the pounds melt away. The three, easy-to-pronounce words are: "No, thank you". Disappointed? Most people are. But the results won't disappoint you. This simple formula (which admittedly requires Spartan willpower), when applied to a passing box of chocolates over a period of time has remarkable results.'

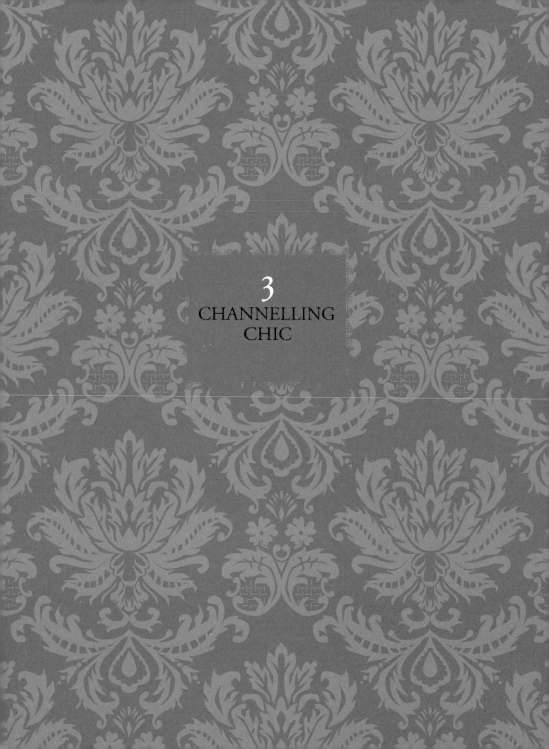

3
CHANNELLING CHIC

CHANNELLING CHIC

You've compared your body type with the string-limbed skinniness of Audrey Hepburn, the broad-shouldered athleticism of Katharine Hepburn through to the well upholstered curves of Sophia Loren. You've read and ignored their dietary advice. Now it's time to steal their style! Audrey, Marilyn, Victoria Beckham and Kylie Minogue developed the perfect formulas for dressing to suit their bodies and by doing so provide fantastic templates for our personal use.

In this chapter you will learn how to dress like your star shape using the tried and tested principles of the world's most fabulous women. Marilyn Monroe, for instance, dressed to show off her voluptuousness, rather than attempting to disguise it, and favoured halternecks as a result. Femme fatale Marlene Dietrich drew attention away from a bosom she felt was rather soft by showing off a fantastic pair of legs. At the 1951 Oscars ceremony she walked up the stairs to present an award in a dress split to the thigh.

Audrey Hepburn's advice? Work out what suits the proportions of your body and stick to it rather than following the whims and dictates of catwalk fashion. That way you may even find yourself creating trends rather than following them. Remember that stars today have personal stylists but those in the past didn't and had to find their individuality through a process of trial and error.

Fashion
FADES, ONLY *style*
ENDURES.

Coco Chanel

Audrey Hepburn had a passion for fashion, confessing that 'some people dream of having a big swimming pool – with me it's closets.' It was all about understated style. Her cool combination of a wool pea-coat with slim jeans was adopted by that other fashion maven Jackie O, while at night Hepburn, and modern Ballerina Nicole Kidman prove you can never go wrong with a classic sleeveless LBD.

BALLERINA MUST-HAVES

➤ A WHITE COTTON SHIRT that will act as a flattering spotlight on your face. Gap produce good quality classics that won't break the bank.

➤ SEVEN-EIGHTHS JEANS that are skinny and stop just above the ankle. Be sure to wear them with ballet flats for true Audrey style.

➤ A CASHMERE WRAP, Audrey's was a discreet navy and went with her whilst travelling.

➤ A BLACK WOOL TURTLENECK and a pencil skirt or black skinny jeans for that *Funny Face* '50's Beatnik chic.

➤ A V-NECK SWEATER WORN BACKWARDS to create a new area of erotic interest – so much more understated than showing off a cleavage you might not necessarily have!

➤ A SELECTION OF SLEEVELESS TOPS to show your toned arms and shoulderblades – if it gets chilly, cover up with a pure wool twin-set.

✹ RIGHT: You don't have to stick with an LBD if you're a Ballerina. Nicole Kidman rocks a contemporary equivalent, the Little White Dress.

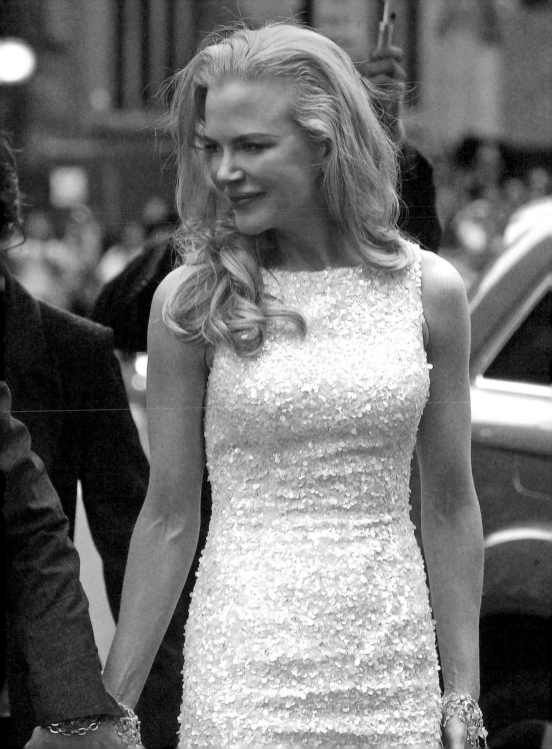

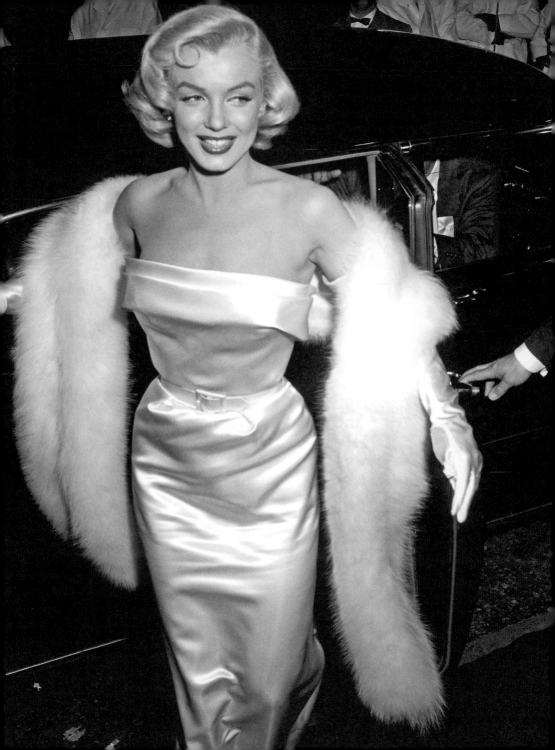

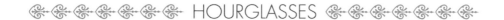

HOURGLASSES

Marilyn Monroe and Sophia Loren had curves that were adorable assets in the war of the sexes! With this body type it's all about looking drop dead gorgeous and devastatingly sexy. In 1953, for instance, Marilyn made an infamous entrance at the *Photoplay* magazine awards ceremony in a gold gown designed by Travila that was so tightly fitted she had to be sewn into it. One male onlooker observed,

'WHEN SHE *wiggled* THROUGH THE AUDIENCE TO COME UP TO THE PODIUM, HER *derriere* LOOKED LIKE *two puppies* FIGHTING UNDER A SILK SHEET.'

Joan Crawford was furious (probably at having her spotlight stolen) and wrote, 'It was like a burlesque show. The audience yelled and shouted … but those of us in the industry just shuddered. Sex plays a tremendously important part in every person's life. People are interested in it, intrigued with it. But they don't like to see it flaunted in their faces.' Marilyn kept flaunting away though in her own inimitable style and Sophia Loren was canny enough to borrow the same dress for a European photo session.

✻ LEFT: Marilyn arrives at a movie premiere in 1954 in a strapless white satin dress and white fur stole to match her white-blonde hair — pure va-va voom!

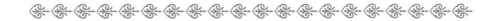

HOURGLASS MUST-HAVES

➤ A TIGHT SWEATER, preferably pastel pink angora. Marilyn followed the Sweater Girl trend in the '50s, so-called because the combination of pencil skirt, tight sweater and whirlpool bra was so alluring. Marilyn wore these tactile tops with tight knee length skirts or white shorts.

➤ A BLOUSE KNOTTED AT THE WAIST to show off the midriff – a red gingham shirt and rolled-up jeans is a good 'at home' outfit.

➤ HALTERNECK SUNDRESSES WITH FULL SKIRTS. They'll give an instant '50s Hourglass effect, especially in polka dot. The halterneck gives the illusion of lengthening the shoulderline and so balances out the hips. Actress Kelly Brook is adept at channelling this look.

➤ A FORM-FITTING WOOL JERSEY DAY DRESS in sand, black or white – Marilyn had several of these button-through belted dresses that she wore with suede high heels.

➤ A PINK SATIN, STRAPLESS, SKIN-TIGHT EVENING GOWN with matching elbow length evening gloves, a.k.a. the 'Diamonds are a Girl's Best Friend' dress. Madonna paid homage to this look (back when she had curves) in her 'Material Girl' video. This style of dress is a fashion classic and is usually found in black, but pink can crop up, too. Look for '50s inspired fashions on the web, such as at poshgirlvintage.com

➤ AN ALL WHITE OUTFIT. This was Sophia's favourite colour because it offset her Mediterranean olive complexion – she had a penchant for wearing a white shirt and matching dirndl accessorized with huge gold gypsy earrings. You don't have to buy real gold, rolled gold is significantly cheaper and gives exactly the same effect.

Those with bodies like Liz Hurley and Victoria Beckham are lucky enough to have ranges actually designed by their prototypes from which to choose. Liz Hurley's beachwear can be bought via elizabethhurley.com and Victoria entered the fashion arena in 2008 with a collection of long and lean dresses following her personal mantra of 'dress sexily, but not in an obvious way'. Both tend to keep shapes slim and simple and the tops tight to emphasize their bust and boyish hips.

BALCONY MUST-HAVES

➤ BOOTCUT WHITE JEANS as worn by Hurley. Her own label does the St Tropez, a pair in cotton with a little stretch for fit, but at £165 they're not for the fainthearted, and keeping them white is a tough call.

➤ A SLEEK KNIT SUIT in sand or cream by American label St John. Angelina Jolie models for this once conservative brand that specializes in elegant separates such as pencil skirts and classic trenches.

➤ FLY-EYE SUNGLASSES to hide from the paparazzi. Victoria does her own DVB range but this oversized style can be bought anywhere from airport concessions right down to your local market or thrift store.

➤ BLOCK COLOURS – Victoria and Elizabeth are rarely seen in prints, while Angelina appears to have an entirely monochromatic wardrobe.

➤ A STATEMENT EVENING GOWN – a plunge neckline, bias-cut, white satin column or a Swarovski crystal-encrusted number in a jewel-bright colour from Dolce & Gabbana or Versace.

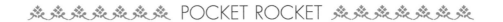

Study the visual delight that is Kylie Minogue. She has moved from being a 1980s fashion casualty dressed in grease-stained overalls as Charlene the mechanic in *Neighbours* to become one of the best-dressed women in the world. Whether gussied up in a crystal-encrusted corset by John Galliano or down in jeans, boots and Belstaff jacket, Kylie is prepared to make statements and has found a look that manages to be both adorably sexy and bang on trend. In 2007 the Victoria & Albert Museum devoted an exhibition to her changing image and stage outfits that, despite a rather snooty reception from the British press, broke box office records.

Another Pocket Rocket, Elizabeth Taylor was no slouch in the fashion stakes either, by her early twenties she owned more than a hundred dresses, 80 belts, 40 cardigans and a full-length mink coat. At the age of 60 she was spotted in skin-tight black jeans, a leather jacket and rhinestone-encrusted cowboy boots. Taylor continues to be an inspiration for the world's top designers including Michael Kors, who admits 'there's a little Elizabeth Taylor in every collection I do. For spring 2005 we had a white dress with an empire waist and some turquoise and jet crystal on it. It was a perfect La Liz moment. For spring 2006 everything was based on the movie *Giant*. Sometimes when I'm working, I use shorthand and say something like, "You know, it's an Elizabeth Taylor *BUtterfield 8* moment!"'

POCKET ROCKET MUST-HAVES

➤ SILK SHANTUNG KNEE-LENGTH COCKTAIL DRESSES in honey, amber or electric blue – a key Liz Taylor look.

➤ HOT PANTS. One of Elizabeth Taylor's finest sartorial moments saw her entering Heathrow airport in a pair of tiny white hot pants with a crocheted trim and matching cut-out kinky boots. Husband Richard Burton paled into insignificance beside her.

➤ A DRESS THAT HAS A NIPPED-IN WAIST AND A SWEETHEART NECKLINE, as worn by Taylor in *A Place in the Sun* (1951) and designed by Edith Head. The heart shape of this neckline displays the shoulders and cleavage to amazing effect without being too provocative.

➤ A SHORT BAT-WING SLEEVED, CLOSE-FITTING JUMPER DRESS. This 80s inspired look is a cover-up that remains sexy yet the only thing you are showing off is your perfect pins. Kylie knew she had to be formal but still star shaped when she went to Buckingham Palace to accept her OBE for services to music in 2008. As she put it,

'THIS IS *incredible* BUT, BEING A WOMAN, THE *second* THING THAT COMES TO MIND AFTER "THIS IS *amazing!*' IS "WHAT WILL I *wear?*"'

So I chose to wear something not too over the top.' Kylie plumped for Yves Saint Laurent, a dress in luxe cream satin embellished with multi-coloured sequin stars plus a pair of Jimmy Choo Lance sandals in gold metallic leather and a mirrored 4½" heel – and she negotiated the gravelled entrance entirely successfully.

Super Sloane Princess Diana, ice maiden Grace Kelly and tomboy Katharine Hepburn exemplify athletic dressing at its finest. Diana's height was an essential component of her look, with legs that writer Julie Burchill described as 'express ways to delirium'. Her Royal Highness cleverly combined all the key elements of athlete style – backless dresses by Bruce Oldfield in black velvet to set off her porcelain skin, one-shouldered ivory satin gowns covered in tubular-shaped bugle beads by Catherine Walker and Cleric that highlighted her strong swimmer's shoulders, and bright bolero jackets that showed off her sinuous frame to full effect (and disguised her lack of waist). Her finest sartorial moment was in response to Prince Charles revealing his adultery with Camilla Parker-Bowles on British TV in 1994. The night it aired she unfurled herself from the back of a black limousine and strode through a parade of flashbulbs to the *Vanity Fair* annual fundraising event at the Serpentine Gallery in London in an off-the-shoulder black chiffon mini dress by Christina Stambolian with a cleverly designed floating waist panel. The finishing touch? A pair of high black silk Manolos and siren red nail varnish. Camilla who?

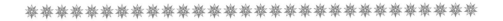

ATHLETE MUST-HAVES

➤ REVITALIZED CLASSICS. Designer Joanna Sykes is perfect as she combines a modern androgyny with a feminine sensibility in her white silk T-shirts, cigarette-cut leather jeans and black wool trousers with a flattering high waist and flat front. Stockists include the celebrated Matches boutique, now online at matchesfashion.com.

➤ DELUXE SPORTSWEAR – these are the shapes in which you are most comfortable. Look out for Sophie Hulme (sophiehulme.com), who plays with classics like the bomber jacket, which she covers in silver or night blue sequins. For less extreme pieces seek out brands like Adidas that collaborate with designers Yohji Yamamoto and Stella McCartney.

➤ THE ENTIRE WARDROBE DESIGNED BY ANN ROTH and worn by Jane Fonda as Bree Daniels in the classic 70s movie *Klute*. Fonda's outfits include a high-necked, low-backed, black sequinned evening sheath with long sleeves; a high-necked micro mini dress worn with a low-slung, big buckled belt covered up with a mini trench and thigh-length boots; and singlets worn with a high-waisted midi skirt.

➤ A BLACK TUXEDO channelling Yves Saint Laurent's iconic *le smoking*, the first tailored trouser suit designed for women based on men's evening wear. Be inspired by the 1970s, an era in which YSL, Bianca Jagger, Andy Warhol and Liza Minnelli hung out at infamous New York disco Studio 54 in a whirlwind of strobe-lit high gloss glamour. If you can't afford a real *le smoking*, go to a classic men's outfitters such as Moss Bros or the evening section of Marks & Spencer, which specializes in classic pieces. Like Bianca, who wore a white tuxedo on her wedding to Mick Jagger, wear nothing underneath for instant adorability.

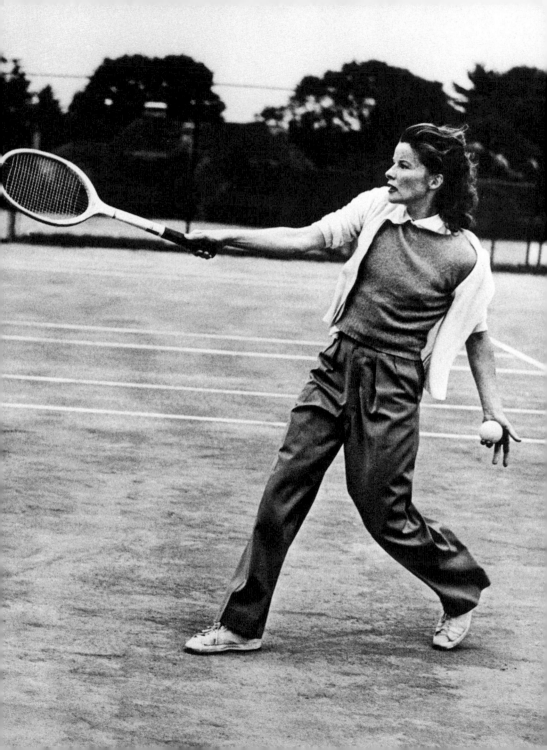

Why I Wear Trousers
by Katharine Hepburn

Katharine Hepburn was one of the first
women in America to wear trousers
habitually, considered a subversive act
in the 1930s because they signified a
woman who had independence from a
man. They defined her as an individual
within the Hollywood system and
became a source of press interest that
heightened her allure. A popular gossip
columnist, Jimmie Fidler, headed up
one article with the question, 'Why do
you wear pants?' She answered 'They
are comfortable and convenient. And
because it seems to amaze people. I like
to do unusual things.'

✹ LEFT: Katharine Hepburn was an athlete fully aware of
her body's physicality. She dressed in an easy slouchy style
that has come to exemplify American chic.

Big girls can be bombshells! Take heed of Mae West, the Empress of Sex, as she was dubbed in prewar Hollywood. The daughter of a boxer and a corset model, she rose to fame after her self-penned hit *Sex* was banned from Broadway in 1926. The resulting publicity catapulted her into the upper echelons of film stardom and she relished roles in which she played a sexual aggressor as persistent as any man. Her most famous line, 'Why don't you come up and see me sometime?' was directed at Cary Grant in the movie *She Done Him Wrong* (1933). At her first meeting with costume designer Walter Plunkett she entered the room in ten-inch platform shoes, a foot-high blonde wig and ... nothing else, saying,

'*Honey*, I THOUGHT YOU'D LIKE TO SEE THE *beautiful body* YOU'RE GONNA HAVE THE *opportunity* OF DRESSIN'.'

Diane Brill, one of the top models of the 1990s and a muse for catwalk designer Thierry Mugler, channels Mae West today. Measuring 43–29–43, Brill seemed a fertility goddess in a fashion world dominated by the waif-like body of Kate Moss. She said, 'You have to feel that your uniqueness makes you superior. Simply feel secure in the knowledge that what you've got is special and deserving of adoration. Only if you have the strength of this conviction will you have the great guys of the world eating out of your hand.'

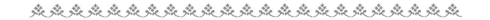

BIG IS BEAUTIFUL MUST-HAVES

➤ A CORSET TOP. Whatever your size, you need to create a waist and *anyone* can do this with a corset. Vollers create the best, a company with a pedigree that stretches back to 1899 when it operated under the name Madame Voller. Its corsets are made-to-measure, hand finished and available in a vast range of sizes online at vollers-corsets.com. Dress up with a long black evening skirt and show off the lovely soft skin of your shoulders and cleavage.

➤ DON'T WEAR ANYTHING THAT LOOKS AS IF YOU'RE TRYING TO HIDE. Diane Brill banned anything baggy from her wardrobe, saying, 'No sacks, no Moroccan tents, no colossal kaftans. Best on big women: well-tailored suits, impeccably cut dresses.'

➤ BE INVENTIVE – if you can't find what you want, make it or customize an existing garment. Follow Diane Brill's 'destroy to create' theory by reconstructing vintage clothes. She used to take apart an entire man's suit and remake it, turning the jacket double-breasted, adding leather trim, overdying the fabric, pleating the trousers, and fastening leather D-ring buckles to peg the legs.

➤ A SMART SIDE IN COMEBACKS. As Mae said, 'I never worry about diets. The only carrots that interest me are the number of carats in a diamond.' If asked whether you've lost weight, say, 'No, it's just shifted around a little.'

How to Create a Trademark

The remarkable thing about fashion today is that there is so much room for individuality. The rules of dressing are more relaxed than ever before – so why do so many women look the same with their skinny jeans, tango tans, Ugg boots and GHD straightened hair? The greatest stars of stage, screen and the fashion catwalk know that making a statement makes a girl stand out from the crowd of this season's homogenized blondes and gives a special brand of appeal.

Gloria Swanson, the grande dame of 1930s film, fused forever on celluloid in her comeback movie *Sunset Boulevard* (1950) always carried a single red carnation and her left arm always sported a selection of thick gold slave bracelets. Marion Preminger, wife of the director Otto, always made an entrance in the 1950s by stopping dead at the top of a flight of steps. She then let her white mink stole drape to the floor while dragging it slowly off with one hand.

One 1950s movie star, Kathleen Hughes, appeared at the fashionable Dem Mar beach club in California wearing polka dot toenails to match her red and white polka dot dress. Today Victoria Beckham often sports an Hermès Birkin bag in an identical shade to her dress, and Kate Moss combines bedhead tousled hair with a pair of shades and skinny legs accentuated by drainpipe jeans or a mini. As the celebrated Hollywood costume designer Edith Head once said, 'Having a consistent look means something to the public.'

Certain trademark looks take more commitment than others though. In July 2008 Victoria Beckham had just settled down to a lengthy flight from Los Angeles to London. With her face free of make-up she snuggled down in the airline-issue pyjamas. Suddenly the plane was brought to an emergency stop, halting just before take-off as a stray bird was sucked into the engine and a small fire broke out. Rather than panicking, Victoria calmly stayed aboard after other passengers had left, painstakingly reapplying her make-up and donning her designer clothes to look picture perfect when changing planes.

Some trademarks are natural, and what is often perceived as a handicap at the start of a star's career can prove a blessing. Both Gloria Swanson and 1980s supermodel Cindy Crawford had a prominent mole on their face, and on her first *Vogue* cover Crawford's was digitally removed. It later became so closely associated with her that she starred in a series of adverts for chocolates in which she was seen to accidentally flick her mole off her upper lip. Vivien Leigh had large hands so amassed a collection of 150 pairs of gloves to cover them.

If you don't have a natural trademark, develop or invent one – the way you wear your hair, an unusual piece of jewellery like a vintage charm bracelet or super-sized cocktail ring. Show your wit with a Lulu Guinness or Billy Boy handbag in the shape of a fan or floral basket, and be aware that you can sometimes come across both these designers' wares in TK Maxx!

Don't Look Like a Celebrity, Look Like a Star!

The difference between a celebrity and a star is obvious. A true star doesn't need to look as if she's tried too much (even if hours have been spent to achieve that effect). Paris Hilton is a celebrity, Kim Novak is a star. Follow these basic rules:

➤ NEVER show cleavage and legs at the same time. If a hint of breast is on display, your legs should be covered. Pamela Anderson always shows both and she is clearly a celebrity as a result. Adorable star Gwen Stefani displays a refreshingly old-school attitude to her very contemporary look, believing that 'to me a little bit of sexy – a heel – is plenty sexy. You don't have to give it away in the first few seconds.'

➤ Just one word, TANOREXIA. Having day-glo orange skin is never glamorous. You should remain as God intended or go for a Californian sun-kissed look like Grace Kelly or Jennifer Aniston.

➤ NO Juicy Couture jogging suits – that's the difference between Jenny from the block and the diva that is Jennifer Lopez.

➤ Bubblegum pink is for CHEERLEADERS and Paris Hilton – intense pinks are worn by adorable women. The most glamorous shade is 'shocking' pink introduced by 1930s couturier Elsa Schiaparelli in a collection of clothes designed to complement the colour of a 17.47 carat pink diamond, known as the Ram's Head, sported by one of her best clients and queen of the European social scene, Daisy Fellowes. (Daisy also wore Schiaparelli's iconic Shoe hat, made of black suede and with a bright pink heel, it took the shape of a shoe worn upside down on the head.)

➤ NO T-shirts with slogans, unless they are vintage and pre-1982. NEVER, ever wear a T-shirt of a seminal rock concert that you never went to. In some of her least glamorous moments Kate Moss took to wearing T-shirts emblazoned with The Clash, a band that was at its height when she was in her nappies.

➤ NO hair extensions.

➤ NEVER go out without wearing panties. The only person who could get away with this was Marilyn Monroe.

➤ DON'T swig out of a bottle or a can – your drink should always be in a glass, hopefully with an olive. DON'T over-indulge either, that is for glamour model wannabes on cheap package holidays to Playa de las Americas. It is NEVER glamorous to eat the Tequila worm.

➤ DON'T be caught smoking on camera unless the cigarette is in a holder (see Audrey Hepburn as Holly Golightly in *Breakfast at Tiffany's*).

➤ NO open-mouthed kissing in public.

➤ DON'T bare your breasts in public. It's OK if it's in a tasteful pin-up but NOT in the full glare of the paparazzi. And if a topless shot of you emerges, shake it off with aplomb like Marilyn Monroe. An old calendar shot taken when she was desperate for work was discovered in 1952 just as she was beginning her stellar advance to the top. Asked by a reporter if she had anything on, she replied, 'Oh yes. I had the radio on.'

➤ ONLY smooch other girls if you mean it.

➤ A lady NEVER kisses and tells.

➤ NEVER date a footballer, they may be as rich as Croesus but they will make you look cheap.

➤ NEVER, ever make a sex tape – this can never be glamorous. As Bette Davis said, 'Glamour is so mysterious and fragile. It's a fascination with the unknown. But how is glamour possible when you know everything there is to know about celebrities? Now we know what they look like without their clothes, who they're sleeping with, everything!'

➤ DON'T act stupid when you're not. As Reese Witherspoon said,

'CREATING A CULTURAL ICON OUT OF SOMEONE WHO GOES, "I'M *stupid*, ISN'T IT *cute?*" MAKES ME WANT TO *throw daggers*. I WANT TO SAY TO THEM, "MY GRANDMA DID *not* FIGHT FOR WHAT SHE FOUGHT FOR JUST SO *you* CAN START TELLING WOMEN IT'S *fun* TO BE *stupid*. SAYING THAT TO YOUNG WOMEN, LITTLE GIRLS, MY *daughter?* IT'S *not* OK.'

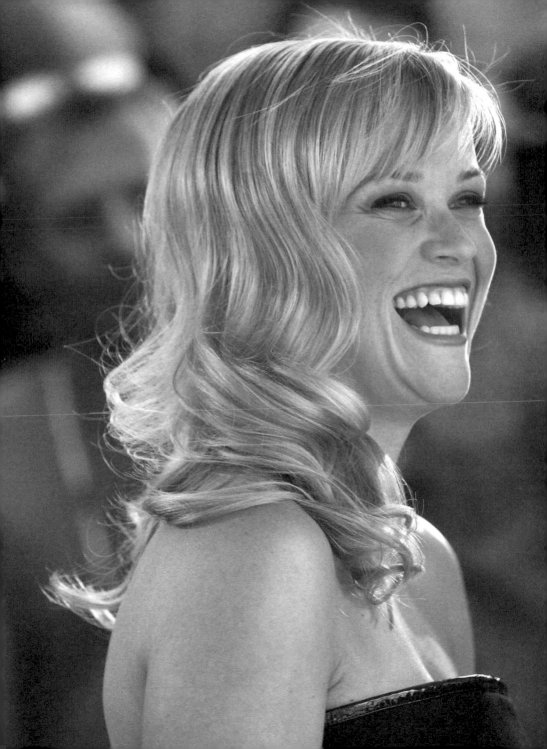

Individuality *leads to Invention*

Movie star Joan Crawford once admitted, 'I feel that clothes are people. When I buy a dress, that's a new friend. Am I to let it hang there and not give it warmth and affection? Course not!' Crawford, like many of us, was a fashion addict but she took it to obsessive extremes, sometimes changing her clothes up to ten times a day – she was even said to have a special outfit for signing her fan mail. She once asked Clark Gable to take her to see a play in Los Angeles. He said, 'But you've already seen the play.' She replied, 'Yes, but not in this dress.'

Joan Crawford was 5'4" with small flat hips and huge shoulders. Frills and bows were out for her and from the 1930s onwards, in collaboration with the Hollywood fashion designer Adrian, she accentuated her look with shoulder pads and pencil skirts – a basic fashion formula she adopted until her death and one that was copied by women all over the world. It became a 1940s fashion trend and has undergone revival after revival ever since, most notably in the catwalk collections of maverick British designer Alexander McQueen. By ignoring fashionable trends and concentrating on an individual style Crawford created rather than followed fashion. Agyness Deyn has done the same today, almost single-handedly kick-starting the early 1980s post-punk revival with her prom dresses and peroxide locks be it a modern quiff or a deconstructed bob.

IF YOU *want*
TO SEE THE GIRL NEXT
DOOR, *go* NEXT DOOR.

Joan Crawford

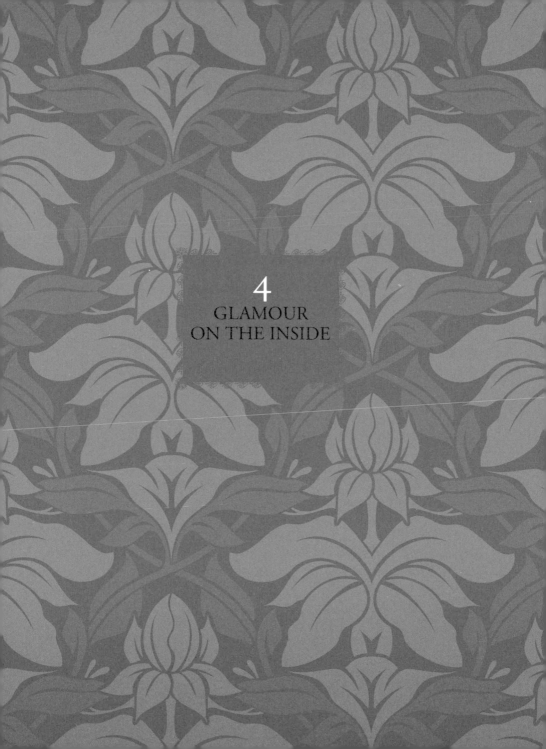

4
GLAMOUR
ON THE INSIDE

GLAMOUR ON THE INSIDE

Glamour isn't just about having the right handbag – it's about having the right personality too and some of the world's most adorable women have been gorgeous inside as well as out. Irene Dunne managed to be one of the most famous film stars of the 1930s as well as a woman who was adored by those around her. She was never rude, even to the most intrusive of journalists – her strategy was to appear gracious, a little vague and always polite while rapidly heading to the nearest exit. She had a number of loyal friends including screen idol Douglas Fairbanks Junior and was happily married to her only husband, a dentist, for 37 years. Unlike stars today (stand up Lindsay Lohan!) there were no reports of her 'difficult' behaviour or of being led off a set due to 'emotional distress', and she never checked into rehab. She charmed everyone she met and was known to be a loyal and steadfast friend.

The same can be said of other iconic stars, who continue to be much loved presences on the modern stage and screen. Jackie O may have been elegant and sophisticated but we want to *be* Audrey Hepburn; Naomi Campbell makes heads turn but we'd sooner spend an evening with Erin O'Connor. This is because these women have warm personalities as well as good looks and never give the impression of stabbing others in the back to get to the top.

Flattery Will Get You Everywhere!
by Arlene Dahl (1965)

❧ The easiest way to earn a compliment is to give one. When you tell a man you like his tie, rave about his rumba, or praise him on his putting, he is bound to recognise you as a woman of rare taste, charm and discernment!

❧ Let people know that you think they're wonderful.

❧ Never upstage – don't top people's jokes, even if you have to bite your tongue.

❧ Never launch loudly into your own opinions on a subject – whether it's petunias or politics.

How to have an
Adorable Personality

Irene is a perfect example of how it's not enough to look gorgeous – you have to fine-tune your personality too. *Charm* is the key to gaining glamour on the inside, it's the invisible part of beauty – and nobody who is devoid of charm can be truly divine. A sparkle in the eye that glints as if you are keeping a saucy secret to yourself, a mouth that turns up instead of down, a sense of humour and love of life will draw people to you. If that's combined with a knowledge of what's going on in the world, a keen interest in others and an air of relaxed confidence, you'll be the belle of the ball.

Doyenne of romantic literature and step-grandmother to Princess Diana, Dame Barbara Cartland was an expert on charm – so much so that she wrote a book on the subject in 1965. As she put it, 'you can't expect charm to fall on you like manna from heaven. Whatever charm you had in infancy has probably disappeared – and in any event retention of babyish charm into adult life would be artificial and incongruous. A good many women attempt this – and very uncharming they are as a result. Spurious charm can be found everywhere. The simpering film star, the grinning TV advertiser, the flirtatious male hairdresser. They probably antagonize as many people as they entice!'

DO

➺ BE GOOD AT LISTENING, convey a genuine interest in what people around you say – have the gift of 'wanting to know', as Barbara Cartland put it.

➺ REMEMBER BIRTHDAYS and write thank you notes.

➺ BE COURTEOUS. Mean it when you ask someone how they are!

➺ BE POLITE – these days stars can get away with nothing, even giving inadequate tips. Check out stainedapron.com for a list of the best and worst celebrity tippers fresh from the mouths of waiters, plus inside stories on their manners (or lack of!)

➺ DON'T LAUGH AT ANOTHER PERSON'S MISTAKES. Queen Victoria was entertaining at a formal state dinner. As the dessert loomed, finger bowls were brought in to a visiting foreign potentate. He drained it in one gulp. To prevent any social embarrassment, the Queen picked up her own finger bowl and pretended to relish the contents!

➺ BE PREPARED TO LAUGH AT YOUR OWN. In 2005 Halle Berry won the Golden Raspberry for Worst Actress, an award given as an inverted Oscar each year to celebrate the most heinous performances rather than the best. Usually winners ignore the accolade but Berry not only turned up at the ceremony to accept her Razzie, she gave a hilarious eight minute acceptance speech which ended 'if you can't be a good loser, you can't be a good winner.' Her sense of humour meant she was unanimously lauded as a woman of true class.

→ GIVE OUT COMPLIMENTS and accept them with good grace.

→ KEEP EYE CONTACT. If you look away when someone is talking to you, they will think you are bored and you'll be in danger of being labelled a Cocktail Cuckoo! Dame Barbara Cartland coined the phrase to describe, 'a social figure who always looks over the shoulder of the person they are talking to – apparently in an effort to see if anyone more important is present! I call those sort of people the Cocktail Cuckoos because they are always searching for a bigger and better nest!'

→ BE RELAXED. Gloria Swanson swore by standing on her head every day to eliminate tension, as did Arlene Dahl, who had a portable slant board in her office on which she lay at an angle for 20 minutes every morning. You could make one yourself using an ironing board propped up at a 30 degree angle at one end! Just lie down on it with your feet up, it apparently promotes the circulation of the blood and does wonders for the hair follicles as well as destressing you after a hard day at work.

→ JUST BE NICE! Take heed of film star Dolores del Rio's wise words, 'Every bad deed, every bad fault will show on your face' – so start being nice before the wind changes and you're stuck with that pout for ever! Smile when you look people in the eye and you will be surprised how many people will smile back – it's an automatic response that will help set the mood of every encounter.

→ NASTINESS IS BEST AVOIDED. Today's celebrities know they can get column inches if they call each other out. Paris Hilton and Nicole Richie have been sniping at each other for years for supposedly stealing each other's thunder. Jewellery designer Jade Jagger and Kate Moss also famously fell out when Jade discovered that Kate was sleeping with her boyfriend Dan Macmillan behind her back. Her revenge – she sent Kate a beautiful diamond studded necklace in the shape of the word, 'Slag'. But these antics are more akin to playground pigtail tugging than the work of grown women. It takes the Grand Guignol feuding of stars of the past to put it in its proper perspective.

The most infamous Hollywood enemies were Bette Davis and Joan Crawford, who were pitched head to head for decades as the most ego driven queens of the silver screen. Bette conducted her war with words – Joan with deeds, which usually involved stealing Bette's man. At Bette's first important press conference Joan crashed in with her new husband Donald Fairbanks Junior dressed to the nines and looking fabulous. All eyes turned to her and Bette was forgotten. Bette retaliated with *bon mots* such as, 'There goes the original good time that was had by all' and,

'JOAN SLEPT WITH *every* MALE STAR
AT MGM *except* LASSIE.'

Their famous feud came to a head during the filming of *Whatever Happened to Baby Jane* in 1962. In one scene a silver salver was lifted by Joan to reveal a dead rat placed there by a malevolent Bette – Joan screamed and fell in a dead faint. To get her own back Joan wore a heavy weightlifter's belt in a scene where Bette had to carry her across a room. Bette did it in one take and then screamed in agony as her back went into spasm.

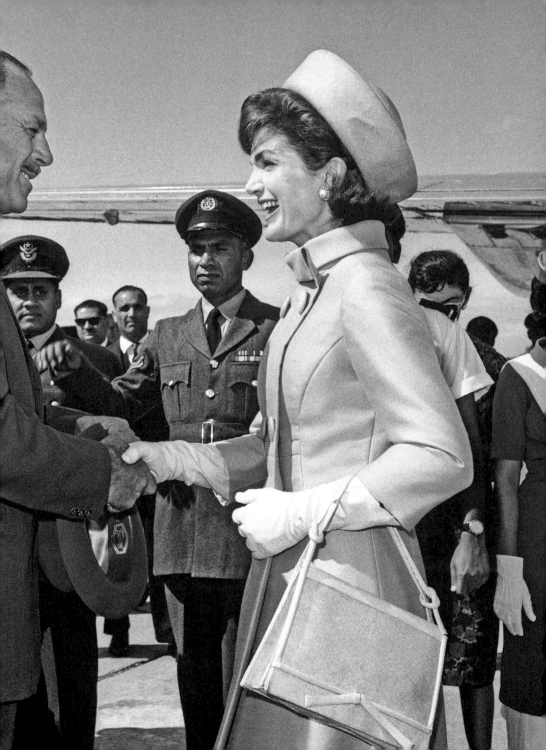

Conversational Charm
in a Capsule

It's not just what you say – it's the way that you say it. Jackie O would speak so softly that men would have to lean in close to her to follow her every word and fix their gaze on her soft peach coloured lips. Audrey Hepburn was said by admirers to pronounce every word as if she caressed it in a lovely modulated tone. Cecil Beaton said of her voice, 'With its unaccustomed rhythm and sing-song cadence that develops into a flat drawl ending in a childlike query, it has the quality of heartbreak.' Film director Peter Bogdanovich called it 'purred elegance'. Jane Fonda charts her development from a mere girl into a rounded, complete human being by listening to her own voice in her early movies. She found it moved from being adolescent, high and thin to her well-known husky tone when she was in *Klute* and 'beginning to inhabit myself as a woman'.

✳ LEFT: Men were mesmerised by Jackie O's breathy little girl voice. Her erudite knowledge of art history and interior design only added to the adorable mix.

How to Speak Like
Grace Kelly

In all her movies Grace Kelly had a voice of incredible elegance – charming, mellifluous and subtly sexy. But it wasn't always like that! Her rather harsh Philadelphian accent belied her patrician good looks and *had* to be changed if she was going to become a successful model and actress. In the 1950s Grace was snapped up by John Robert Powers, who had founded his Powers model agency in New York in 1923 – it went on to become one of the fashion industry's most successful. Women dreamed of becoming one of the Powers Girls and his alumni included Lucille Ball and Ava Gardner.

A successful Powers Girl had personality as well as poise and had to follow specially developed programmes of improvement in order to be transformed from top to toe. One that was particularly pertinent to Grace was the voice modulation and diction programme reproduced here in its entirety so you can learn to speak just like her!

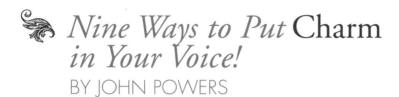

Nine Ways to Put Charm *in Your Voice!*

BY JOHN POWERS

1 BE ENTHUSIASTIC. Put happy words in your speech, words that express enthusiasm. Say them with a tone that expresses your enthusiasm:

> Thank you for a *wonderful* evening
> It was such a *grand* party
> What an *interesting* collection
> We *enjoyed* having you
> Yes, I'd *love* to come

Practise hanging on for an extra second to the words that reveal your enthusiasm.

2 PUT A SMILE IN YOUR VOICE. A smile can be heard as well as seen. The next time you speak on the telephone arrange to sit near a mirror so you can see whether your smile is there. If you smile as you speak, the smile will be reflected in your tone. Don't forget to hold the happy words to emphasize them. And smile as you read such sentences as these aloud:

> I am *so* happy to hear about your new job. Congratulations and *good luck*!

3 KEEP MONOTONY OUT OF YOUR VOICE. Read this sentence without changing your tone level:

I SAW THE NEW ART EXHIBIT AT THE MUSEUM TODAY.
• •

Now try the same sentence following these dips and rises:

I SAW THE NEW ART EXHIBIT AT THE MUSEUM TODAY.

Notice how a dull statement of fact becomes an interesting report. Lead upward to the important words in order to give your voice variety and emphasis. A monotone makes your listener lose interest, no matter how exciting your story. Start off with a normal lowered tone so you can rise without straining or forcing your voice.

4 DON'T SPEAK IN A SHRILL VOICE. Since the female voice is naturally higher pitched than a man's, it gets out of control more easily. A shrill voice grates on the nerves and indicates tension and strain. Work to bring it down to a pleasing, lower pitch. Your posture affects the sound of your voice. Raise your ribcage to give your voice room to get out. When your chin is resting on your chest, your voice has to fight to escape. Keep your head high and level to prevent constriction of the throat muscles and vocal cords.

5 DEVELOP RESONANCE IN YOUR VOICE. Speaking through pursed lips, clenched teeth and locked jaw stifles the resonance. Practise talking with a relaxed lip and jaw action. Test the difference by whispering across the room. To make a whisper understood at a distance calls for exaggerated mouth action. You won't want to keep up the exaggeration in public, but it is a good private means of practising resonance. Open your mouth properly when you speak and let the sound flow out in deep, rich tones.

6 TAKE YOUR TIME. Don't rush through your words. Slow down the pace and you will sound more confident, less strained. Open your mouth and move your lips while speaking. It will slow you down and make you easier to understand. If you're in a hurry to finish what you're saying, your listener will be equally eager to have you finish. Create interest in your conversation by speaking in an easy, relaxed manner.

7 SPEAK CLEARLY. Clear speech is well groomed speech. Don't be careless about slipping over your consonants. L and R are often overlooked. Hold those letters and say them clearly:

Instead of *awright, awready, awmost*, roll out the L and say *all* right, *all* ready, *all* most – Instead of sistuh, brothuh, mothuh, say sister, brother, mother.

8 AVOID A NASAL TWANG. N, M, and NG are the nasal sounds. They must vibrate through the nasal passages to have a pleasant sound. When they are voiced through the mouth rather than the nose, they are distorted and have an unpleasant twang. Remember when you've had a bad head cold and your pronounciation of M, N and NG couldn't get through the stuffed nasal tract?

Pinch your nostrils closed and say hum, none, some, come. Feel the stifled vibrations? Now release the nostrils and hold the M and N sounds. Hummmmm, nonnnne, sommmme, commme. Do the same with NG: sing, ring, cling, wing. Release the nostrils and hold the NG sounds: singi*ng*, ringi*ng*, clingi*ng*, wingi*ng*. Always let these three important nasal consonants come forth in a pleasant, low pitched tone.

9 CONTROL THE VOLUME OF YOUR VOICE. A loud voice is not becoming to a lady, and a loud voice becomes a shrill voice. Have you ever listened to the sounds of women's voices at a large party? As the talk becomes more animated, the voice pitch rises until it is almost deafening. Lower your volume and you will lower your pitch. If your articulation is perfect, you can be heard clearly even though your tone is soft.

How to Change Tack

If the skeletons in the closet are rattling so hard they're waking up the whole street, have no fear. Take charge and change tack! Carla Bruni's image revamp gives hope to all – one night she goes to sleep as a model cum singer-songwriter and wakes up several hours later as the First Lady of France, adored not just in France but all over the world. Her change of tack has made her stand on the world's stage as the new Jackie O, complete with the same bandbox neat style and selection of chic pillbox hats. And if we examine Carla's change of tack, who knows, it could help us on our way to Parisan power brunches, bed and breakfast at Buck House and head-to-toe Dior.

Carla started off as a model working in an industry famed for its drug-fuelled debauchery, temper tantrums and egomania, a pretty unsuitable background for a woman who has since become a global ambassador for France. Independence was her motivation – and for this we adore her, particularly as she cites feminist independence as the main factor in her career choice. Carla says, 'it is a major duty for women to be independent. Independence was my obsession when I was 20. It was not making money; it was making my own money. Modelling meant I did not have to rely on my parents or a man.' She cites Simone de Beauvoir's famous feminist tract *The Second Sex* as a major influence.

In 1997 Carla changed tack, leaving the world of modelling for a major rebrand as a singer-songwriter. Her first album was produced by an ex-boyfriend, Louis Bertignac, the accompanying videos directed by another ex, Leos Carax (notice a pattern here?). Her husky vocals and breathy delivery were adorable – who could resist? It sold two million copies. So follow Carla's example and stay friends with your boyfriends, you never know when they will come in useful!

Carla has never been afraid to date an unlikely Adonis, even men considerably shorter than her – another adorable quality. It must have helped a little that she met her husband Nicolas Sarkozy at a dinner party when they were both seated, allowing their *coup de foudre* to flourish at first on an intellectual level. Now she wears flats whenever with him in public. It's not all been one way though – Carla has been good for his image, too. Prior to marrying her, Nicolas was dubbed 'President Bling-Bling' for his somewhat flashy style. Carla persuaded him to swap his flashy gold Rolex for a chic Patek Philippe.

When you become a public figure, former life comes back to haunt you – that's a given. Carla has had well-publicized affairs with a number of famous men, including Eric Clapton and Mick Jagger, and once said,

'I BORE MYSELF SILLY WITH *monogamy.*
I PREFER *polygamy* AND *polyandry.*'

One of her most adorable aspects is her insouciance about her past lovers and sexually freewheeling past, saying, 'It's not that I've had lots of lovers. It's that I never hide them' and on Jagger, 'I don't know what the fuss is about – there are 7,000 girls.' And the nude shots that surfaced on the internet? 'I have a body that would allow me to pose nude without being provocative.' Pure class!

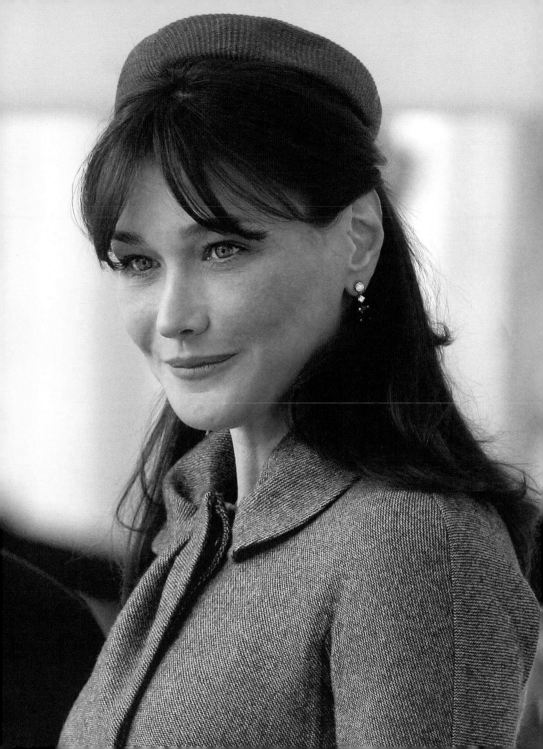

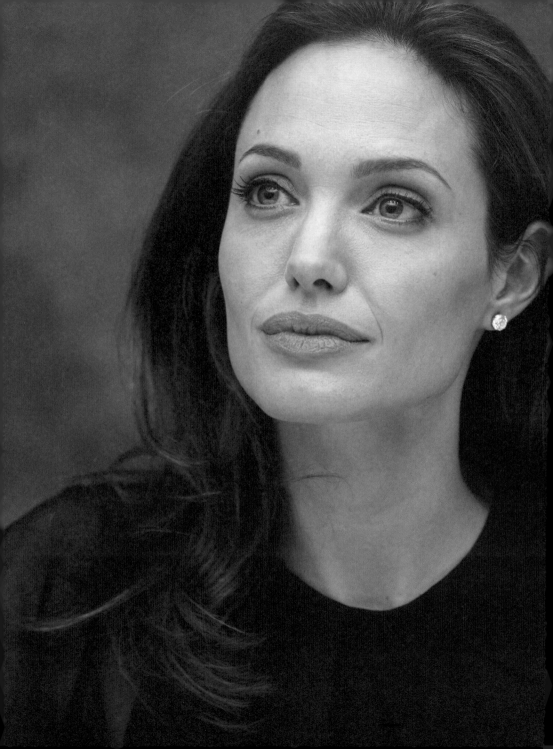

How to be a Humanitarian Like Angelina Jolie

The greatest Hollywood glamourpusses have good looks and great clothes, kindness, intelligence, sincerity and charm. Without these attributes they would be mere mannequins. But there is one magical ingredient left – a charitable heart.

IRENE DUNNE was a delegate to the United Nations and a foundation in her name raised $20 million for St John's Hospital in Santa Monica, California. She also adopted a four-year-old girl, Missy, from the New York Foundling Hospital. On her death at the age of 92 in 1990, President Ronald Reagan said, 'Losing her is like losing a member of the family. She's a special lady who will live in our hearts for ever.'

ELIZABETH TAYLOR adopted a baby who had been born prematurely in Mering, Germany with a congenital hip injury that needed extensive and expensive corrective surgery. Elizabeth described their first meeting: 'The German officials wanted me to have "a perfect baby". I had to fight like a tiger to get her. To me she was perfect. She was covered with abscesses, suffering from malnutrition, had a hip that was going to cripple her for life – and I just loved her. She didn't cry and she didn't laugh. She watched everything and I held her and I bathed her and I changed her for three days and finally she started giggling. This funny little introverted person that was just sort of half asleep responded so much to love – the warmth, I think, of two arms. I was hooked by the end of a few days. Her first word was "Mama". I guess it's universal, but when it happens you just die.'

✴ LEFT: Angelina Jolie is famed today, it seems, less for her film roles than her large brood of children and her countless humanitarian causes.

After the loss of some of her closest friends to the illness, Elizabeth Taylor became one of Hollywood's first AIDS activists saying, 'I felt early on that people needed to be better educated about the disease. I just couldn't sit back and watch this terrible sickness take so many of my friends without wondering if there was something I could do.' In 1985 Taylor established a national AIDS foundation to fund scientific research and organised a Commitment to Life dinner that raised a million dollars. In 1991 she founded the Elizabeth Taylor AIDS Foundation, which has been responsible for raising at least $8 million for distribution to HIV/AIDS foundations around the world (to make a donation, visit elizabethtayloraidsfoundation.org).

Today ANGELINA JOLIE, a celebrity with a clear-cut social conscience, is a goodwill ambassador for the UN High Commisioner for Refugees – a role that has led to her visiting at least 15 war torn countries including Sudan, Darfur and Chad and personally donating millions of dollars. Angelina has also become mother to several biological and adopted children – including Maddox, found in a Cambodian orphanage in 2002, Ethiopian Zahara and Pax from Vietnam. Once a wild child but now a doting mother and dedicated campaigner, she has no problem aligning her past and present:

'I'VE BEEN *reckless*, BUT I'M NOT A *rebel* WITHOUT A CAUSE.'

Angelina is a shining example but the rest of us have to begin our good works a little more slowly. What about these ideas for starters?

→ Think about changing your credit cards so that a percentage of any money you have spent on a purchase goes to charity – once it's done you don't even have to think about it!

→ Use the web browser goodsearch.com. It's a search engine that donates 50 per cent of its revenue to more than 45,000 charities.

→ Shop with igive.com – up to 26 per cent of each purchase goes to charity.

→ Donate your frequent flyer miles to the Make a Wish Foundation – donate.wish.org/donate/miles. It takes children with life threatening illnesses on dream holidays abroad and needs at least 2.5 billion air miles per year.

→ Make the most of any opportunity to give and remember that charity donations are tax deductible! You can make online donations at charitychoice.co.uk, a website that has links to thousands of different causes that need your support.

→ Join VSO (Voluntary Service Overseas), which has been in existence since 1958 to fight global poverty and disadvantage. You could take a career break from two months to two years and find yourself in China, Bangladesh or Papua New Guinea. Visit vso.org.uk for more details.

Famous and
Fabulous *Friendships*

Hollywood may not seem the kind of place that fosters long-lasting friendships, especially when many girls are up for the same roles in such a cut-throat business – but you'd be surprised! Jennifer Aniston and Courteney Cox have been best buddies since meeting on the set of *Friends* in 1990 and Courteney is always there when Jennifer needs a shoulder to cry on after another disastrous date. (The pair have an unbreakable tradition of dining every Christmas Eve at Mastro's of Beverly Hills, a classic Rat Pack era steakhouse at 246 N Canyon Drive). Jennifer says, 'You can tell a girl's girl from a mile away. Courteney's not stand-offish, she's not threatened by women, and she doesn't have to throw her womanliness all over you to show you what kind of woman she is. She's comfortable and that makes you feel comfortable.'

Katharine Hepburn was married to Ludlow Ogden Smith but her primary relationships were always with women, such as Laura Harding. As she put it, 'I think men and women are more shut off from each other than a woman and a woman.' Drew Barrymore and Cameron Diaz famously share 'jazz' cigarettes together, and Kate Moss, Sadie Frost and Davinia Taylor, a.k.a. the Primrose Hill Set regularly meet for Sunday roast at Club Kitchen, Davinia's basement kitchen in her house in St John's Wood, London. Hairdresser James Brown, a long time friend of Moss describes the group as 'always giggly, like little girls. It's not a bitchy crew: we've all been friends for a long time. It's like the Waltons, the psychedelic Waltons. Everyone really gets on.'

✳ ✳ ✳ ✳ ✳ ✳ BE A BEST FRIEND ✳ ✳ ✳ ✳ ✳ ✳

➤ IT TAKES TIME to be a best friend – it doesn't just happen overnight but you should *recognize* a potential friend in an instant. As Davinia Taylor puts it, 'You kind of click and that's that. Like goes to like.'

➤ BEST FRIENDS TALK AND LISTEN to one another equally – at any time of the day or night. Marlene Dietrich nailed it when she said, 'It's the one you call at 4am that really matters.' 'Constant use will not wear thin the fabric of friendship' wrote Dorothy Parker.

➤ BEST FRIENDS ARE LOYAL and can trust each other with their secrets. As the Ancient Greek philosopher Euripides wrote, 'One loyal friend is worth two thousand relatives.'

➤ BE THERE – even if you wish you were somewhere else. Friends come first.

➤ STAND BY YOUR BEST FRIEND when everyone else fades away. Surveying the maelstrom of her personal life, Elizabeth Taylor said, 'You find out who your real friends are when you're involved in a scandal.'

➤ TELL THE TRUTH and expect it in return, even if it's painful. As Cher said, 'I can trust my friends. These people force me to examine myself, encourage me to grow.' A best friend is someone who knows you and loves you just the same!

➤ And as Gwyneth Paltrow says,

'THE *best* WAY TO MEND A BROKEN HEART IS *time* AND *girlfriends*!'

How to Develop a Radiant *Expression*

Looking appealing is pleasing to others, pursing your lips like a cat's rear-end or scowling like a bulldog chewing a wasp is not. Victoria Beckham would gain a lot more fans if she stopped pouting like a prima donna but insists she doesn't do it purposefully,

> 'WHEN I SEE PICTURES, I DO SOMETIMES THINK, "*You miserable cow!*" BUT IT'S JUST THE WAY MY FACE FALLS.'

Victoria, like many others, could make herself look beautiful by simply changing expression – an impossibility for today's frozen-faced stars. The scourge of Botox is so rife that seeing a genuine life-enhancing grin on the red carpet or runway is as rare as the proverbial hen's teeth. Red blooded women are being replaced with identikits, faces formed of immobile slabs of unlined orange flesh. So ditch the Restylane, banish the botulinum toxin A and smile, smile, smile – and if you've forgotten how, John Powers can remind you:

'Skim through the pages of any glossy magazine and study the faces of the models. What makes you pause over the girl at the wheel of a new car, sipping a soft drink or smoking a cigarette? Her features are good, yes. But the quality that grasps and holds your attention is the model's radiant expression. These girls can't afford to let a petty annoyance rob them of that look of glowing happiness when they face the camera's eye. Yet how many women let unpleasant thoughts and carry-over reactions destroy their facial radiance when they face the eyes of their friends, families and business associates. By consciously training your face to wear an attractive expression, you will be taking a giant step up the ladder of beauty.

- Keep the corners of your mouth turned upward as much as possible. Even when you're listening to or discussing a serious subject, there's no need for the mouth to take a downward droop. The down lines are ageing lines. Learn to avoid them.

- Smiles are habit forming. What's more, they are contagious. People are searching for happiness. They will naturally gravitate towards a woman who looks happy.

- Don't wear a foolish grin like a clown's painted mouth. The happy look springs from the eyes as well. Don't be a deadpan. Let your face mirror your pleasure.'

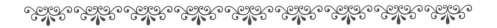

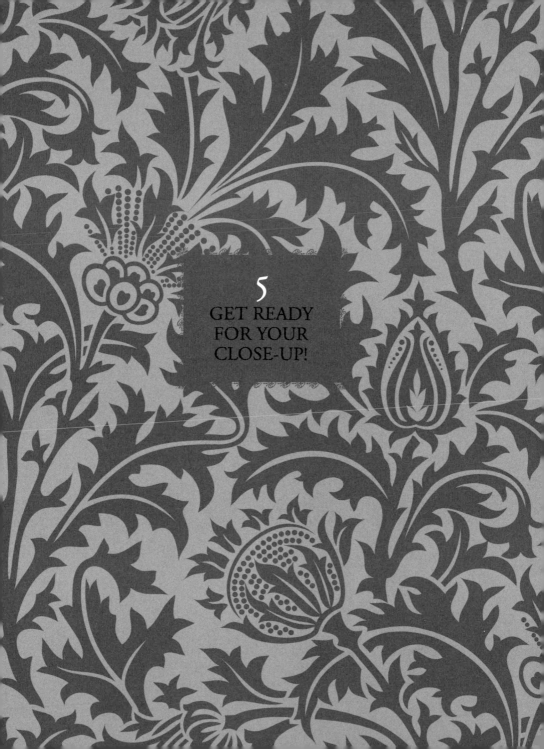

5
GET READY
FOR YOUR
CLOSE-UP!

GET READY FOR YOUR CLOSE-UP!

A slash of red lipstick, a hint of blush on a cheekbone and a lick of coal black mascara are essential weapons for today's fashion battlefield – no wonder we call make-up war paint! Glamourpusses of the past were quick to recognize this, even the understated Audrey Hepburn admitted to 'a lot of help from Estée Lauder' and stayed true to the same make-up team of Alberto and Grazia de Rossi throughout her career. Marlene Dietrich evocatively described her relationship with her cosmetician as that of 'accomplices in crime' and Ann Sheridan, when feeling down, summoned her make-up man with the words, 'come over and put some oomph on me!' Lana Turner was so aghast at her personal make-up artist being drafted into the army just before she was due to start filming *The Postman Always Rings Twice* (1946) that she persuaded him to teach her all his tricks so she could do her make-up for the film herself. She felt unable to trust anyone else with her perfect visage.

Hollywood make-up artists were privy to many of the stars' greatest secrets and knew how to turn the ugliest ducklings into the most soignée of swans – careers soared sky high when the right make-up was applied. After her top-to-toe Hollywood make-over Marlene Dietrich, once just a plump cabaret singer from Berlin, became one of the most potent seductresses on celluloid, as did Greta Garbo, a heavy-browed melancholy Swede who was transformed into

'The Face' by Gustaf Norrin. Some stars refused their proposed make-up changes, though, insisting on keeping the physiognomy they were born with, including Lauren Bacall, who was sent to Perc Westmore, head of the make-up department at Warner Brothers before her first screen test. After examining her face, he recommended plucking her thick and angular eyebrows, shaving her hairline and straightening her teeth – she refused and her idiosyncrasies made her a star.

The movie maven with the most control over her own image has to be Claudette Colbert. Hollywood glamourpuss and perfectionist to the extreme, Colbert became totally obsessed with how her face looked on film after a make-up artist told her that she photographed best on her left side. From that moment on she made sure that in every movie the entire right half of her face (or 'the dark side of the moon' as one director called it) was covered with a lurid green greasepaint so that it could never appear in shot. At the height of her success in the 1930s after starring in *It Happened One Night* (1934) with Clark Gable she ordered an entire set to be rebuilt because the position of one doorway meant that she would be entering from her wrong side. As a result film crews nicknamed her the 'Fretting Frog'.

❧ *Top Tips from* Hollywood's Greatest *Make-Up Man!*

Harry Meret the esteemed make-up director at RKO in the 1950s, put together a list of essential make-up dos and don'ts. They remain as useful today as ever.

❅ DO give some thought to the colour of your dress before applying your lipstick. You may look stunning with vivid orange lipstick but, please, don't use it when you wear a red dress. And never select your lipstick because the colour looked well on someone else.

❅ DO sharpen your eyebrow pencil to a chisel edge. That is the secret of a beautiful brow. Use a razor blade for the sharpening – and use it often. Of course, short fine strokes create a natural effect. After the pencil, brush your brow gently with an old toothbrush to soften the line.

❅ DON'T use rouge, unless you are exceptionally pale. Rouge is misused so often that I believe it's safest to stay away from it entirely – particularly blondes. Create your own natural glow with proper skincare.

❅ DON'T use coloured eyeshadow in the daytime. This looks garish and tasteless. To accent your eyes in the daytime, line the lid near the lashes with soft brown pencil and apply a little mascara. That's all you need.

HOW TO
Make-Up Like Marilyn

Marilyn Monroe had a classic bombshell look that became her trademark. It's an easy look to copy – all you need is red lipstick, black liquid liner, mascara, taupe and matte white or silver eyeshadow, eyebrow pencil, mascara and blusher.

And before you start the step-by-step guide listen to her words of advice: 'Study your face very carefully to decide what features you want to focus attention on. No man likes a girl whose face looks like a piece of fancily decorated pastry, but if you're careful you can even bring up the heavy guns like eyeshadow and he'll never know you're "made-up" at all! In my view most girls look more desirable with glistening lids and a moist mouth. A drop of oil on the lids will give the effect, and if you're handy with a lipstick brush there's nothing like it for that luscious look.'

1 A thick, arched, well-groomed eyebrow is essential if you want to look like Marilyn. You may need to fill yours in with a tawny brown or taupe eyebrow pencil or shadow and then set it in place with a clear gel.

2 Carefully blend smooth matte liquid foundation all over your face using a soft damp sponge.

3 Photographer Eve Arnold said that Marilyn's greatest asset was her translucent white, luminous skin. To get this effect use MAC Strobe cream (maccosmetics.com), a new generation highlighter that can be worn over or mixed with your foundation. Apply it lightly over your cheeks – its translucent and pearlised qualities will give you Marilyn's shimmering glow.

4 Clearly define the eyelid's crease with a brown or charcoal powder eyeshadow and apply a little lightly under the eye.

5 Use a matte white or pale pink eyeshadow as a base on your eyelids – Yeyo Powder White by Urban Decay (urbandecay.com) is perfect for this. Completely cover the eyelid, making sure you take it into the inside corners.

6 Use the same eyeshadow to highlight the browbone.

7 Line the upper lash line with a black liquid eyeliner as close to the lashes as possible. Make sure the line tapers from thin to thick in the middle and then to thin again. Sweep the line up and out towards the browbone. No lash line is needed underneath.

8 Fake the eyelashes. Marilyn's were applied only halfway across the top eyelid. You can buy eyelashes in this length. Alternatively, just cut a false eyelash in half. Your false eyelash should begin in the middle of your eye and end at the outer corner.

9 Curl your lashes and apply two coats of mascara from base to tip on the top lashes only, then a much lighter coat on the bottom lashes. Remember – the emphasis should always be on the top of the eyes.

10 Your secret weapon is Bobbi Brown Tinted Eye Brightener (bobbibrowncosmetics.com) applied to the outer corners of the eye. If you take it up at an angle, it will hide any drooping Margaret Thatcher effect!

11 Using a circular motion, apply some pink blush to the apples of your cheeks with a big brush.

12 Use a lip brush to cover your lips with a matte red crème lipstick. (For the best true red, see The Daring Dozen on page 117). Cover with some clear lip gloss or for true Marilyn effect use her trademark Vaseline.

13 The last and most important step – use a black eye pencil to create Marilyn's beauty spot on the left side of your face, just above your lip.

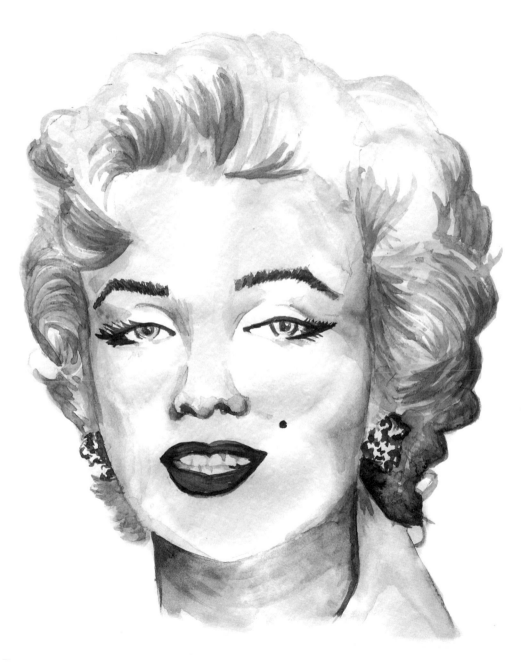

HOW TO GET
Marlene Dietrich's *Cheekbones*

Marlene Dietrich is said to have had her molars taken out
to give herself more defined cheekbones (although she
vehemently denied this) and used to suck on lemons between
takes to keep her mouth and cheeks taut. You don't have to
go that far – even the roundest of face shapes can get a bit of
Marlene definition with the right contouring techniques.

1 Take a medium-sized brush and some blusher that
matches your skin tone.

2 Find your cheekbones – the simplest way is to take two
fingers and locate the bone where it starts by the centre of
the ear and follow it down. The secret is to apply the blush
underneath your cheekbones (in what's usually referred to
as the hollow of your cheeks).

3 Use your brush to follow the hollow under the bone
until you have a '70s-looking stripe on both cheeks.

4 Then take a big brush and blend in using an up-and-
down motion (not backwards and forwards or you'll look
like a '70s throwback again.

5 Now apply blusher in a lighter tone over the top of the
bone and blend in so there are no obvious gaps. Voilà –
you now have cheekbones!

✳ RIGHT: Once Marlene Dietrich had located and
exaggerated her cheekbones she changed from a
German hausfrau to Hollywood dynamite.

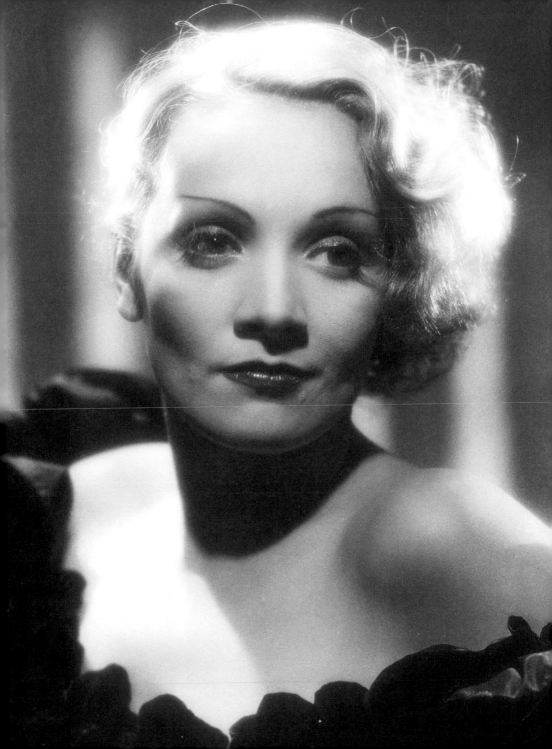

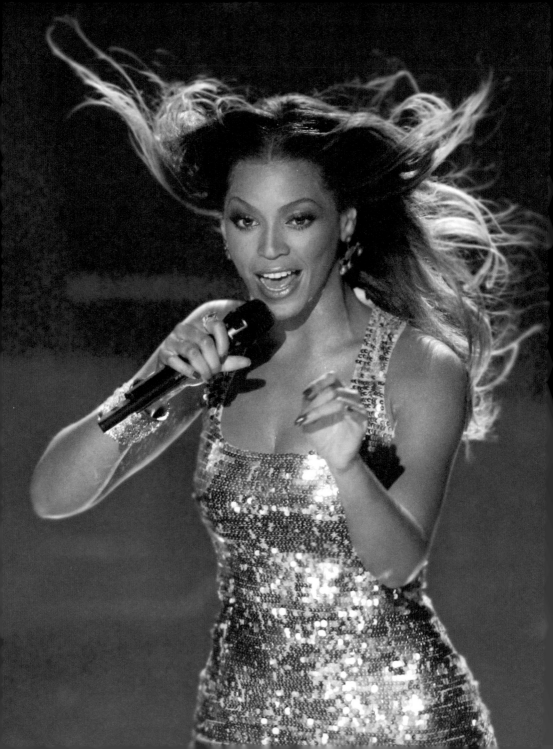

Look Like a Diva – Beyoncé Knowles

➤ The skin of a true R&B diva glows, so use a light-reflecting moisturizer on your face and neck. Apply sheer foundation with a sponge, blending carefully as you go. Then use concealer to cover blemishes or dark shadows under the eyes. Tip – it's important not to use any powder, this look is a shiny, not matte look.

➤ Beyoncé's caramel coloured skin suits a tawny shade of cream blusher that is placed on the apple of the cheek, smoothed upwards and blended over the cheekbone.

➤ The diva look needs a strong brow to balance out that mane of hair, so use a brush of medium brown powder to fill in your natural brow, accentuating the arch as you go.

➤ Beyoncé's amazing feline eyes are emphasized using a clever trick. Pale brown matte eyeshadow is spread over her entire eyelid stopping just under the brow, which is then highlighted with a white shimmer shadow. A black eye pencil is used to circle her eye and then winged out, 1950s-style, at the outer corners. Then the clever part – a metallic gold or silver shadow is applied to the corners of her eyes around the tear ducts – this adds an incredibly intense sparkle that literally lights up the eyes. She finishes off with two coats of black mascara.

➤ If you study Beyoncé at any red carpet event you will immediately notice that she practically always wears a neutral lip colour, usually a nude or pinkish brown gloss.

✻ LEFT: On stage Beyoncé morphs into her alter ego 'Sasha Fierce' whose luscious body has provided a image of life-enhancing femininity for the 2000s.

Lip *Allure*

Since Cleopatra painted her lips a deep carmine to lure the mighty Caesar, lipstick has been the ultimate quick glamour fix – you may not be able to afford Dior catwalk couture but a Dior Addict High Shine in Flamenco Red is within the reach of most pockets. We all love a lipstick and Gwyneth Paltrow has extolled the virtues of a kick-ass red – although it has to be said that her rather thin lipline looks more successfully sexy in pale shades and naturally shaded gloss. Bette Davis was another lipstick obsessive – her shade was famously dubbed 'whorehouse red' by the writer Tennessee Williams and the actress admitted that,

'*Even* WHEN I'M AT HOME *alone*,
I WEAR MY LIPSTICK. I FEEL *naked*
WITHOUT IT.'

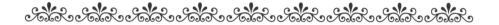

LIPLINES

The most iconic celebrity lips are the most luscious. Angelina Jolie's regularly top polls of the world's sexiest pair – a genetic inheritance that none of us will be able to realistically achieve even with modern techniques of augmentation or a pint of Du Wop's Lip Venom. Joan Crawford's career was in the doldrums after her 1920s flapper image became dated. Then Max Factor invented a lip shape for her that he dubbed 'the Smear', which ran above and below the natural contours of her mouth with just the slightest of bows at the centre top – the brand new shape was later renamed 'the Hunter's Bow'. It was the perfect shape for Joan's rather heavy jaw as it considerably lessened the space between the lower edge of her mouth and the bottom of her chin.

Crawford's revamped lips were show-stopping, huge and glamorously glossy – 'labial flamboyancy' said one critic and 'like balloon tyres in wet weather'. *Marie Claire* magazine urged caution for women thinking of copying this overblown lip look however, unless they could balance it with Crawford's 'hippopotamus eyes'.

Today labial flamboyancy, now known as 'trout pout', has become an unfortunate fact of celebrity life as a result of over-zealous use of lip enhancement. Lindsay Lohan, Britney Spears and Christina Aguilera have all sported suspiciously large porn star lips. If you must indulge remember that the lower lip should be one and a half times the size of the upper lip – if you keep to these proportions your lips should remain looking relatively natural.

Joan Crawford's
Tips for Perfect Lips

* Sit at your dressing table under the brightest light possible – if your make-up looks good here, it would look good anywhere!

* Paint your lips with a brush and the colour will remain longer and smoother.

* Draw a clean outline and fill in boldly.

* Wait a minute, blot with tissue and apply again.

* Or try powdering lightly over the first coat to act as a base for the second.

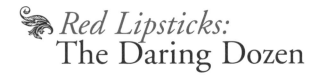

Red Lipsticks:
The Daring Dozen

CLINIQUE DIFFERENT LIPSTICK IN ANGEL RED – a blue toned red as seen on pale faced Nicole Kidman in Moulin Rouge (clinique.com).

MAC COSMETICS LIPSTICK IN RUBY WOO – matte retro red worn by Madonna on her Blonde Ambition tour (maccosmetics.com).

MAC VIVA GLAM suits pale skins like Kate Winslet and Keira Knightley.

CHANEL ROUGE HYDRABASE CRÈME RED – rich and moisturizing.

NARS FIRE DOWN BELOW – a rich matte red (narscosmetics.com).

NARS JUNGLE RED – great for those with olive skin, like supermodel Gisele Bündchen.

MAC SCARLET EMPRESS – a blue red, perfect for pale skins.

MAC RED LIZARD – semi-matte and a true red, perfect for every kind of glamourpuss.

YSL ROUGE PURE NO. 131 OPIUM RED – a classic true red that suits everyone.

MAC RED LIPSTICK IN RUSSIAN RED – as worn by Gwen Stefani.

PALOMA PICASSO'S MON ROUGE – an '80s classic, as worn by Paloma herself. It suits all skin types and dominatrixes with a penchant for Thierry Mugler power suits.

LAURA MERCIER TRULY RED – a lightweight red for lipstick novices. You can apply it in layers until you feel more confident.

✒ *The* Eyes *Have It*

The eyes may be the mirror of the soul, but some adorable stars had nature on their side too. When child star Elizabeth Taylor walked onto the set of her first major movie *Lassie Come Home* in 1943, the director was aghast at the amount of mascara she had on. She was rushed off and her eyes rubbed with a damp towel, but to no avail. To everyone's astonishment she had a double set of eyelashes that surrounded a set of piercing violet eyes.

After Liz the most adorable set of Hollywood peepers belonged to screen legend Bette Davis – there was even a song written about them, *Bette Davis' Eyes* by Kim Carnes in 1981. Bette was said to be able to dilate her eyes for hypnotic effect on screen – as she put it, 'they are the best feature I have to offer the camera.' After her death in 1989, a New York estate auction sold off her effects and a box of her false eyelashes raised the princely sum of $600.

Once eye make-up is on, always remember to take it off, particularly after a hard night on the tiles. You may think sporting panda eyes on the ride to work is rebelliously sexy but you're wrong – you'll look like a raddled reject from Spearmint Rhino. French actress and ethereal beauty Juliette Binoche recommends investing in Lancôme Bi-Facil Non Oily Instant Cleanser for Sensitive Eyes. 'I've used it for over ten years and never changed. I love the fragrance, comfort and efficiency.'

'DO YOU WANT TO KNOW
THE SECRET OF MY SUCCESS?
Easy. BROWN MASCARA, I ALWAYS
BUY *brown* MASCARA. FAIR ACTRESSES
SHOULD *never* WEAR BLACK MASCARA
IF THEY WANT DARK EYES TO SHOW UP.
IT'S THE *opposite* OF WHAT THEY THINK,
THAT BLACK MASCARA WILL MAKE
THEM SHOW UP MORE. OF COURSE,
THERE'S *nothing* LIKE *blue* EYESHADOW
TO SHOW UP BLUE EYES, BUT THAT'S
obvious. THE *secret* IS, IF YOU ARE
FAIR, BLACK MASCARA AND DARK
EYESHADOW WILL MAKE YOU
LOOK LIKE A *clown* OR A *harlot*.'

Bette Davis

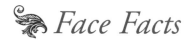 *Face Facts*

Like the shiniest of these stars, you have your own unique face to work with (if not the expertise of their personal make-up artists). There isn't another one like it in the whole world (unless, of course, you have an identical twin). And out of the roughest of raw material can come modern glamour, even if you don't know it just yet!

Jean Kent, one of the most adorable British movie stars of the 1950s, thought that most girls didn't really understand the sheer hard work she put into making herself beautiful. 'If only all the Joans of the world knew the study and care that goes into the grooming and presentation of a film star, they would realize that, if they wanted to look attractive, and were willing to study themselves, the Johns of this world would be worshipping at their feet. The majority of so-called "uninteresting" women can, if they use a little time, and study themselves, find an exciting, rather glamorous woman just waiting for the wrappings to be removed.'

Marilyn Monroe believed that glamour should appear effortless and beauty secrets should be just that – SECRET!

'I NO MORE THINK THAT YOU SHOULD USE A LIPSTICK, POWDER, DEODORANT OR HAIRBRUSH IN *public* THAN YOU WOULD TAKE A *bath* IN PUBLIC.'

Whatever the era, whether yesterday or today, most stars found their own inimitable eye make-up style and stuck with it, barring a little variation when their features began to age. Outside the movie set, Greta Garbo was said by Cecil Beaton to use 'no make-up save a dark line like a symbol on her eyelids – a symbol of no period or fashion, original to our civilization, a symbol which instinct only created.' Audrey Hepburn wore pale lipstick so that all emphasis could be given to her doe eyes, expertly drawn in with liner and mascara. French sex kitten Brigitte Bardot used lashings of black eyeliner liberally winged out at the outside corners, peach lipstick that strayed slightly over her lipline and combined it all with a light St Tropez tan. This routine, said Brigitte, took just five minutes.

'THREE STROKES WITH THE PENCIL, *pif, paf, c'est fini!*'

Go fake though as Brigitte has become the poster girl for the disastrous effects of sun damage! There could be perils along the pathway. Movie star Rosalind Russell had a fantastic tip for perking up a tired face, 'a little make-up tip which at least helps me look alive. I dab a bit of rouge on my temples, just below the hairline.' But a word of caution, 'take care to apply the rouge subtly or you may appear to have a lovely bullet hole in each temple!'

HOW TO GET
Debbie Harry's *Smoky Eyes*

From Bianca Jagger, through Debbie Harry, to Kate Moss today, dark smoky eyes have always been a crucial part of the rock chick look – but today they need to be softer and more sultry than their 1970s and 1980s equivalents. At a shoot for an advertising campaign, the make-up is ramped up to levels that could be a little exaggerated without the accompanying camera, lights and stylist – but an alluring equivalent can be created by you at home. Just follow these few simple steps.

1 Cover each lid with a cream or powder eyeshadow in a dark neutral shade such as deep brown or grey.

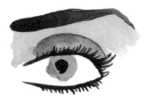

2 Take a darker shade in a toning colour, apply in the eye's crease and blend up towards the corner of the brow. Start with a small amount and then build and blend, checking and rechecking as you go. It's easier to add more colour than take it away!

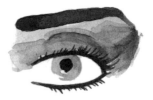

3 Carefully apply black or aubergine eye pencil along the top lashes, smudging with a foam-tipped applicator to soften the line – this is not a 1950s eyeliner

technique with flicked-up corners. Draw the line as close to the lashes as possible, taking it beneath the lashline.

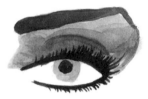

4 Carefully smudge some of the same pencil on the base of the lower lashes, taking it right into the corner of the eye.

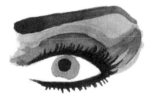

5 Add a small amount of highlight under the eyebrows – but remember, too much is too retro!

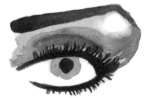

6 Use eyelash curlers on clean lashes, hold for several seconds, and finish the look with lots of layers of luxuriant mascara – top lashes only.

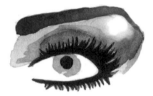

➤ Remember, dark eyes plus a heavy base can look a little dated so try a light reflective base to keep the skin looking fresh and banish imperfections.

➤ The key to successful smoky eyes is to make sure the shadow doesn't slide about as the night progresses. Use an eyeshadow base to hold the colour.

AND ONE LAST TIP
Bianca Jagger used to have a long hot soak in a jasmine-scented bath. She maintained the steam softened her make-up and made it sink into the skin so it lasted longer and gave a mussed-up 'come-to-bed' look.

Elizabeth Taylor's
Perfectly Arched Eyebrows

Cecil Beaton said of Marlene Dietrich, 'Instead of eyebrows, she has limned butterflies' antennae on her forehead.' Marlene, like Jean Harlow and Lana Turner, shaved off her natural eyebrows and substituted an exaggerated pencilled-in arch. Bette Davis' eyebrows were ruined after having been over-plucked at Warner Bros – as she put it, 'I sacrificed two eyebrows for one career.' Ingrid Bergman caused a wholesale change in brow fashion when her natural eyebrows were seen on screen in the film *Intermezzo* in 1939 and Elizabeth Taylor's face was transformed when her brows were plucked into an elegant arch.

Eyebrow shaping is really best left to professionals such as Australia's Sharon-Lee Clarke, whose clients include Kylie Minogue and Julia Roberts. If you get it wrong, you will be stuck with the results for a long time. One of the worst kept celebrity secrets is the Anastasia Brow Studio located in Sephora stores, and Eliza Petrescu (Queen of the Arch), who runs a boutique in her name entirely devoted to eyebrow shaping called Eliza's Eyes located at the Avon Salon & Spa, Trump Tower, New York. Many stars have their eyebrows shaped by Eliza and her minions including Jennifer Lopez and Natasha Richardson, but if you can't afford to pop over to New York many of the biggest stores have their eyebrow experts. Fenwick's, House of Fraser and Harvey Nichols have their own Brow Studios – look out for Shavata, which has branches in London, Edinburgh, Leeds, Manchester and Belfast.

Barbara Stanwyck's Ear
Photoplay April 1935

'The ear is not the most beautiful part of the body, no matter how good it is, but it can be made more appealing and attractive. I like Barbara Stanwyck's ear. It is a cosy intimate ear – the kind a man would like to whisper to, and, she is darn smart to enhance it even more by letting a little curl partly cover it.
So take a tip from Barbara, girls.

'The perfect ear is small and well placed and lies flat to the head. Naturally, if your ear is big and coarse I'll trust you'll cover it with hair – and aren't women lucky they can do that – but any ear is more attractive if it is partly covered and not allowed to flap in the breeze. However, if your ears stick out so you look like a loving cup and sometimes for evening you want to look particularly dressy you can stick your ears back with a little adhesive tape, if you're careful not to let it show.'

How to
Get Rid of a Double Chin
by Jean Kent

'A double chin is the abhorrence of all women.
Stooping over a desk is often the cause so try this
exercise. Throw back the head and bite hard at an
imaginary apple; if done night and morning for a
few minutes, the double chin should disappear. If
the chin is the result of a general plumpness, dust
the fingers and thumbs with talcum powder and,
placing the hands together under the chin, knead
and massage the chin towards the tips of the ears.
Do not use creams. Stroke firmly from the chin to
the base of the throat, and then from the centre
under the chin to the sides. Fifteen minutes a day
should reduce a double chin in a very few weeks but
do remember to keep it up! It is the regular massage
that does the trick and, even though you do think
you have not time, or are too tired, you must be
conscientious. Chin straps are unsightly and do not
make the muscles assert themselves: they merely
push the excessive fat elsewhere.'

HOW TO
Wash Your Face Like
Audrey Hepburn

Audrey Hepburn's skincare routine was low maintenance and minimal – but a with a discreet touch of deluxe. She may have merely washed with soap and water, but the soap she used was anything but ordinary – it was Ernst Laszlo's Sea Mud Soap, which can still be bought today at a mere $39 a pop for 6oz! A solid black cleansing bar fashioned from concentrated minerals from the Dead Sea, Laszlo's was soap fit for the stars, including Jackie O and Doris Day as well as Audrey. The application of Laszlo's soap is highly ritualized:

1 Fill a wash basin with hot water that is comfortable to the touch.

2 Immerse the soap bar in the water and then rub it gently over the face.

3 Dip the soap into the water again and then make a rich lather in the hands.

4 Massage lather over the face.

5 Splash the face 20 times with the basin water, then empty.

6 Splash the face ten times with hot running water.

7 Pat the face dry with a soft towel.

Beauty Confidential

➤ PENÉLOPE CRUZ only uses a light coat of foundation. She uses Teint Innocence Foundation by Chanel in Soft Honey

➤ CAROLE LOMBARD and KIM NOVAK shaded their cleavage lines and lightened the top part of their breasts to make them appear larger.

➤ MARLENE DIETRICH contoured her face with make-up – Jennifer Lopez and Beyoncé use her techniques today.

➤ GLORIA GRAHAME stuffed tissue under her upper lip to give herself a sensuous pout.

➤ BARBARA STANWYCK and LUCILLE BALL pulled loose skin back from their faces using surgical tape hidden under the hairline above the ears.

➤ AUDREY HEPBURN'S make-up artist used to separate each of her eyelashes with a pin after applying mascara.

➤ LUPE VELEZ caused a sensation at the Coconut Grove when she appeared in a gold evening dress and gold evening sandals with gilded eyelashes to match.

➤ MARLENE DIETRICH never used mascara on her lower lashes as she believed it cast a shadow under her eyes.

➤ MARILYN MONROE painted her fingernails with clear polish 'to make them whisper "hold me, hold me"' but painted her toenails bright red, saying, 'I think feet usually aren't pretty, so I use a vivid polish so that they will look saucy.'

✹ RIGHT: Penelope Cruz always favours a dramatic eye over any style of maquillage. She often uses a navy eye-shadow with a smudged navy eye-liner on top.

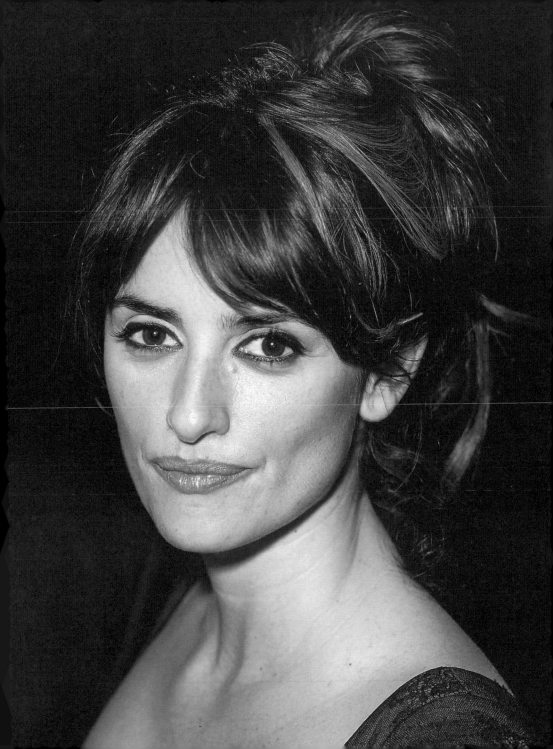

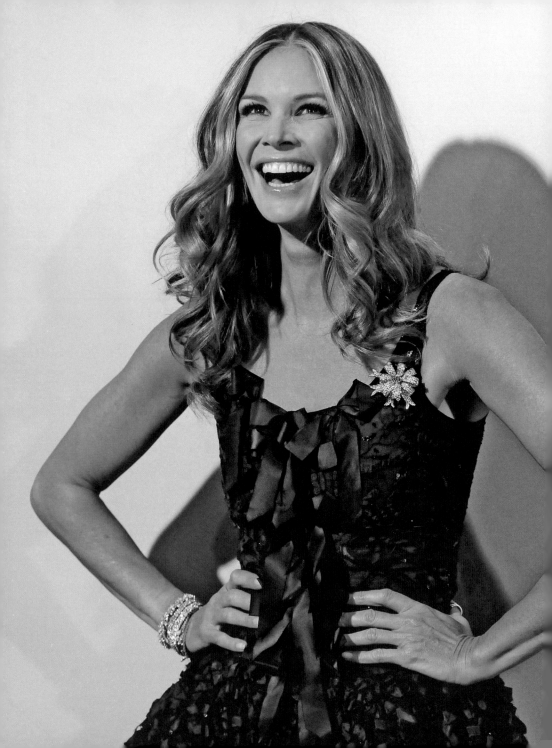

➤ JOAN CRAWFORD chewed gum to firm up her jawline.

➤ BETTE DAVIS said, 'I always massage my face with cold cream, while sitting in a hot bath softened with bath oil. I dry off with a large cotton towel for stimulation, and for daintiness, a brisk rubdown with eau de cologne follows.'

➤ ANGELINA JOLIE is obsessed with body lotion: 'I love to put on a lotion. Sometimes I'll watch TV and go into a lotion trance for an hour. I try to find brands that don't taste bad in case anyone wants to taste me.'

➤ MARILYN MONROE said, 'When a man looks into your eyes, he doesn't like looking into an over-heavy mess of mascara and eyeshadow. On screen, I do have to make-up my eyes considerably but off screen I use eye make-up so that it looks completely natural.'

➤ CATHERINE ZETA-JONES munches strawberries to lighten her teeth. Apparently they contain malic acid, which lightens surface stains!

➤ JEAN KENT was a walking encyclopaedia of beauty tips, including
  ✦ 'Be very careful when you apply make-up to carry it under the chin and down the throat.'
  ✦ 'A merest suspicion of rouge on the tip of the chin is rather attractive.'

➤ And a simple but effective tip from ELLE MACPHERSON:

'WHEN ALL ELSE FAILS – *smile!*'

6

HOLLYWOOD
HAIR, HINTS
AND TINTS

HOLLYWOOD HAIR, HINTS AND TINTS

Marilyn Monroe said that 'in Hollywood a girl's virtue is much less important than her hairdo' and the same is true today. Celebrities can fall out of limos legs akimbo but if their hair is less than perfect they enter a dreaded circle of shame courtesy of the weekly style magazines. We've never forgiven Renée Zellweger for that floppy wedge, Cher for those joke shop wigs and Paris Hilton for … just about everything. Magical moments of yesteryear – Neil Armstrong's moonwalk, Bobby Moore thrusting the World Cup aloft, Bucks Fizz's skirts on *The Eurovision Song Contest* – all pale into insignificance alongside the footage of Britney going into meltdown and shaving her head.

So what is it about hair? It can be our crowning achievement or a skeleton in the photo album, a woven monstrosity perched atop our craniums or a shimmering mane of Rapunzel blondeness fresh from a 1970s Timotei advert. We enter the portals of the hair salon with a frisson of anticipation, only to skulk out crying hot tears of resentment and cringing remorse – or, conversely, bound along the pavement in delight feeling bang on trend.

Joan Crawford got it right when she said,

'I THINK THAT THE MOST *important* THING
A WOMAN CAN HAVE, NEXT TO HER *talent*,
IS HER *hairdresser*.'

Once you have found him or her, you should never let them
go. When Jackie O (then Kennedy) went to Paris on an
official jaunt, she loved the French hairdresser who did her
chignon so much that she smuggled him back home on the
presidential plane. Kate Moss's hairdresser, James Brown, is
her very very best friend (they've even launched a range of
very affordable hair care products together that can be
bought online at boots.com) and Victoria Beckham's career
is charted by her hair change courtesy of session stylist Ben
Cooke. In 2008 when Posh appeared in public to publicize
her new fashion collection, her gamine pixie cut made
headlines across the world and led diva Jennifer Lopez to
gush, 'I was so shocked. I arranged to meet up with her the
day she had it done. She didn't tell me what she was doing,
so I turned up and there she was with this incredibly short
black hair. I was knocked out. I told her she looked like
Audrey Hepburn.' Hepburnesque it may have been, but
what Victoria was really channelling was a haircut that truly
changed the world – Mia Farrow's gamine crop of 1966.

❧ *Top of the* Crops

In a moment of sheer rebellion, Mia cut off her waist-length blonde tresses and created an outrageous crop that caused a global furore. In one fell swoop the actress had transformed herself into a vision of fawn-like vulnerability and her waif look inspired director Roman Polanski to cast her as Rosemary Woodhouse in *Rosemary's Baby* (1968).

To publicize the movie, Polanski invited Vidal Sassoon to Paramount Studios to re-cut Mia's hair surrounded by press photographers for a huge fee of $5,000. As Vidal described it, 'I put a gown around Mia. I picked up my scissors. I made the first cut, feeling now like a high priest at a sacrifice. The first lock of hair had scarcely hit the apron when the press were down from their seats, across the 20 yards to the ropes, over them and on top of us. They weren't just breathing down my neck. They were damn near breaking it. They crowded and pushed, hung out of the rafters and lay on the floor. And all the time I was dancing round that small blonde head.'

It was the perfect cut at the perfect time, as many women had been stuck in a bouffant time warp. Mia's and Victoria's short pixie crops were fresh, youthful alternatives in a world of humdrum hair. Over the years, stars as diversely adorable as Sharon Stone, Winona Ryder, Michelle Williams and Halle Berry have all had the chop. Going from long to short makes everyone look younger – it's an instant facelift. Beware though, for a sharp change of style can bring out the talons of your rivals. When Bette Davis had her hair shorn into the new poodle-cut hairstyle in the 1950s, her rival Joan Crawford said:

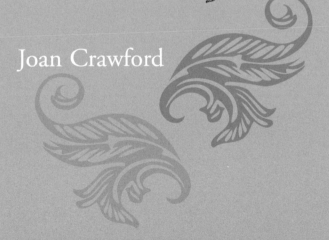

THOSE NEW POODLE HAIR-DOS ARE *not* FOR ELDERLY WOMEN. I THINK THEY LOOK BETTER ON *dogs* AND *teenagers*. I SHOULD KNOW, I HAVE ONE OF EACH.

Joan Crawford

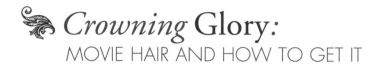

Crowning Glory:
MOVIE HAIR AND HOW TO GET IT

We may not have the resources of Marlene Dietrich, who, when on the set of *The Scarlet Empress* (1932) insisted on having real gold dust sprinkled into her hair so her head glittered under the lights (it cost $60 per ounce, a fortune in those days!) but there are many star hair-dos that are within our impecunious grasps – as well as a few hair-don'ts!

THE LOUISE BROOKS BOB

Louise Brooks in the silent movie *Pandora's Box* (1928) plays Lulu, a flighty young woman who starts as the mistress of a decrepit yet wealthy gentleman and ends on the streets of London as a common prostitute fated to die at the hands of Jack the Ripper. But forget all that! Louise Brooks has the world's most perfect haircut in this film – a glossy black Dutch cut short bob with fringe that has inspired generations of women. The celebrated hairdresser Vidal Sassoon was so inspired by the Brooks bob that he based his seminal 1960s geometric cuts on the look – and Sassoon's is still the place to get the perfect bob today. For your nearest salon visit vidalsassoon.com or ask in your area for a hairdresser who has been Sassoon trained.

THE GRACE KELLY CHIGNON

One way to instant glamour is to put your hair up into a chignon, a name derived from the French *chignon du cou*, which means nape of the neck – where the perfect chignon should reside. Grace Kelly's blonde hair and air of WASP patrician elegance worked perfectly in a chignon. London hair stylist Josh Gibson gives this step-by-step guide:

1 This style works best on hair length that is on or below the shoulder. Ideally, hair should be set first on to rollers to smooth it out (especially if your hair is curly or has a wave) and to help assist in the creation of the shape in the back.

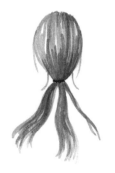

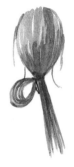

3 Split the hair in the ponytail into two thick sections and one thin one.

5 Smooth out each of the two thick sections with a brush, fold over into a loop and again use a pin to secure to the base of the ponytail.

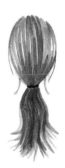

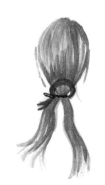

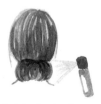

2 Secure hair in a low ponytail either centrally or slightly asymmetrically. Try to tilt the head back when doing this to ensure that the ponytail has an even tension once the head is level again
.

4 Wrap the thin one around the band to hide it, then secure with a pin.

6 To finish the look, spritz hairspray on to the flat surface of a tissue. Wipe this over the head to smooth down any short frizzy hairs.

THE BARDOT BEEHIVE

This look is about tousled bedhead messiness and cries out for a head
of long blonde hair. Set hair on very large rollers to add height and
volume. After removing the rollers, take a medium size section at the
back of the head near to the crown, backcomb, twist and then secure
with a pin just under the occipital bone – if you feel with your fingers
you will be able to tell where it protrudes. Keep adding sections from
both sides of the head, twisting and pinning as you go – the more you
add, and the more you backcomb, the bigger the beehive. Remember
to leave the front sides free to fall mussily over the sides of your face.

For further Gallic inspiration watch *Le Mépris* (1963) directed by
Jean-Luc Godard and you will see the full-on early '60s Brigitte style.
The movie is a bit long-winded so if you can't take any more subtitles
and enigmatic posturing, fast-forward to where Brigitte appears with
a beehive plus thick black headband, shift dress and kitten heels.
C'est magnifique!

'HER BEAUTY AND TALENT ARE *undeniable*,
BUT SHE POSSESSES SOME OTHER, *unknown*
quality WHICH ATTRACTS *idolaters* IN AN
AGE DEPRIVED OF GODS.'

Jean Cocteau on Bardot

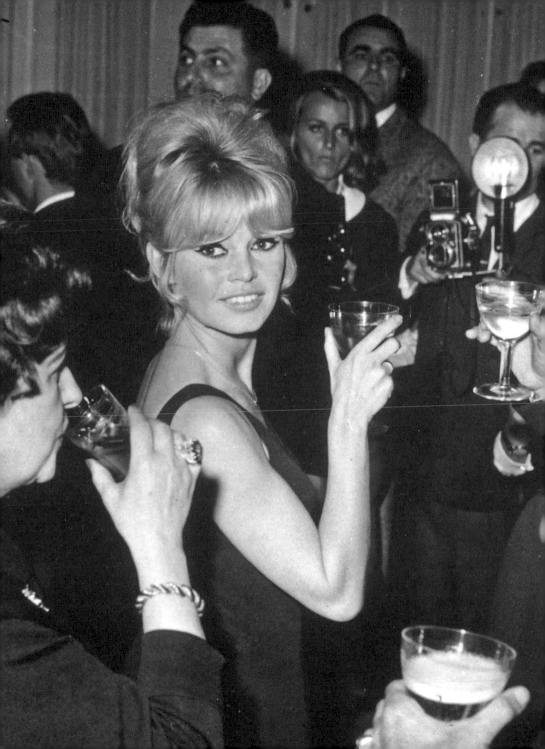

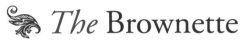 *The* Brownette
– AN ENIGMA BY ARLENE DAHL

'Never underestimate the power of a brownette. She combines the best qualities of blondes, brunettes and redheads. She can be all things to all men. It has been said that gentlemen prefer blondes, rave about redheads, and are bowled over by brunettes – but marry brownettes. The brownette is summer – and a sunny afternoon … roses in full bloom, and a hammock under the trees. She's the all-American girl, the good old summertime, a cloudless blue sky, a gentle breeze, a chocolate soda. She may be a tomboy – or a tease, or a quiet sentimental home girl – but in any case she is a wonderful wife and mother – the girl next door the boys come back to after they've had their fling.'

A modern brownette with full glamourpuss credentials is Spanish actress Penélope Cruz. Her genetic inheritance has blessed her with glossy gorgeous locks but her colourist has also used a clever trick to give her hair a little extra special magic. Wide highlights are placed around the crown of her head in a warm copper tone that is just a little lighter than the overall colour of her hair so she doesn't have that obviously highlighted streaked look. This makes her hair look thicker, a little sun-kissed and super healthy. Ask your stylist to show you how!

It's Fun to be a Redhead

Clara Bow kickstarted a fashion for redheads in the 1920s and actresses Ginger Rogers, Rita Hayworth and Lucille Ball made careers after changing their hair colour to red. Real redheads are rare, less than four per cent of the population – but the good news is that it's the colour that suits most people the best! If you have taken the plunge and decided to go red, remember that red fades more quickly than any other colour so it will be expensive to maintain without the right colourfast products. The best three are:

1 Frederic Fekkai Technician Color Care 3-Minute Mask (fekkai.com)

2 Sassoon Professional Colourprotec Range (sassoon.com)

3 Wella Lifetex Color Protection Conditioning Spray (wella.com)

How to be a Platinum Blonde
by Jean Harlow

Posed suggestively in an Art Deco boudoir, Jean Harlow wore bias-cut evening dresses so tight she couldn't wear underwear and had to bleach her pubic hair to match her incandescently white bob. As film critic Parker Tyler put it, 'Nothing seems to exist between her and her filmy dresses but a little perspiration.'

The first blonde bombshell in Hollywood, Harlow was an overtly sexual film star, known for rubbing her nipples with ice cubes before press conferences to make them stand out, and her risqué repartee with reporters. It was her hair that drew the attention of Arthur Landau, who became her agent after seeing her on a sound stage at Culver City Studios. Bright white and obviously artificial (although Harlow said it was bleached naturally by the sun) it was the beginning of Hollywood's obsession with blondes that continues today. Bright beacons of hair seem to promise uncomplicated fun for men (unless, of course, that blonde happens to be Madonna!). After the release of Harlow's movie *Platinum Blonde* in 1931 sales of peroxide in America soared by a staggering 35 per cent.

Marilyn Monroe remains the most celebrated blonde of the twentieth century and provides a touchstone of inspiration for contemporary stars such as Scarlett Johannson, Christina Aguilera and Gwen Stefani. Naturally a brunette with curly chestnut hair and a penchant for tight sweaters, Monroe was persuaded to go blonde by the formidable Emmeline Snively, owner of the Blue Book modelling agency in Los Angeles. Beautician Sylvia Barnhart of Frank and Joseph's, a movie colony salon, bleached her hair a golden blonde that became progressively whiter as Monroe's career blossomed. The transition to shimmering platinum was affected by Ron Levin while he was working in a tiny suburban salon called Louis and Simone. The owner asked him if he'd like to go in the back and do Marilyn Monroe's hair:

'THERE WAS MARILYN SITTING UNDER THE DRYER WITH HER FEET UP ON FOUR CARTONS OF CLEAN TOWELS, HER GLASS-HEELED CLEAR PLASTIC MULES KICKED OFF, HER BORGANA FAKE FUR DISCARDED, IN A BLACK VERY 1950S POLONECK SWEATER AND TURQUOISE TOREADOR PANTS. AS YOU CAN IMAGINE, I WAS TERRIFIED.'

❧ *Getting* Gwen Stefani's *Hair*

Gwen Stefani is a new generation blonde rock star whose first solo album 'Love Angel Music Baby' shifted millions in 2004. Stefani has had platinum blonde hair since the 1990s – 'I haven't seen my real hair colour since ninth grade' and even wrote a song called *Platinum Blonde Life* for the album 'Rock Steady' in 2001. The Hollywood blonde obsession came full circle when Stefani took on the role of Jean Harlow in Martin Scorsese's *The Aviator* in 2004.

➤ You cannot achieve this level of blonde at home – ignore all those adverts. Peroxide will only get you to a ghastly nicotine yellow.

➤ A professionally trained colourist will show you the secret to white blonde – toner. The toner determines the level of white-blondeness, especially those that contain a touch of blue.

➤ You can't get any degree of hair length if you are platinum – it will quite simply thin out and break off.

➤ Bottle blondes must never swim in a chlorinated pool without wearing a cap – the chemical in the water will turn your hair green. If it happens, douse your hair in tomato juice or ketchup, shower it off and your hair will have returned to blonde.

➤ Being a platinum blonde takes a very high level of commitment and upkeep. Roots need doing regularly and you will need to condition, condition, condition – so, look before you bleach!

※ RIGHT: Gwen Stefani is the latest in a legacy of Hollywood platinum blondes. Hair like this demands incredible upkeep plus augmentation in the form of weft and extensions.

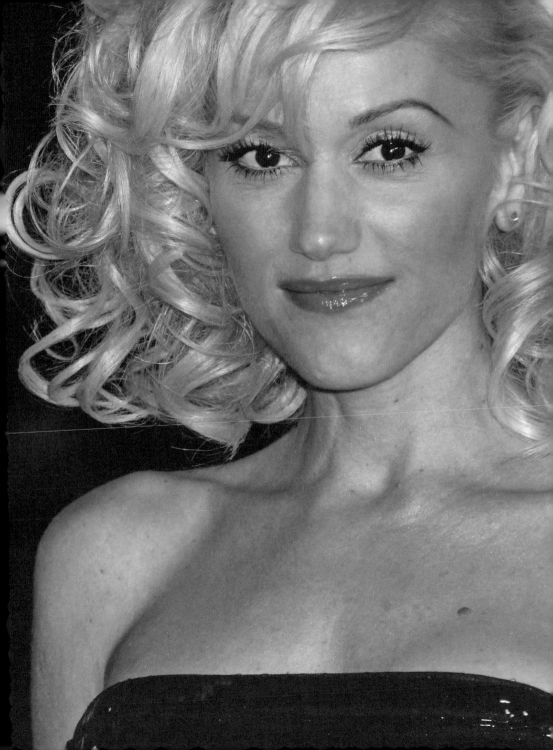

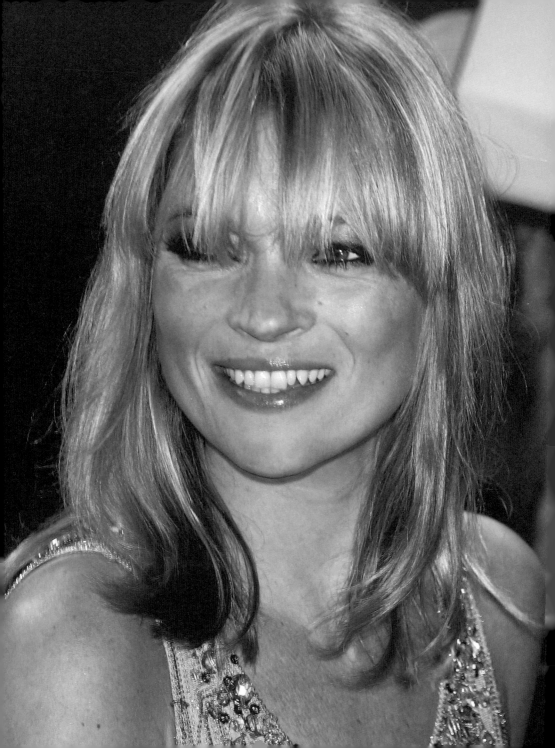

Fringe Benefits: Kate Moss

➤ A fringe suits just about everybody – except those who have the lethal combination of very curly hair and lack of commitment to GHDs.

➤ Some styles are much harder to wear than others. A short fringe like that of 1950s pin-up Bettie Page, for instance, needs confidence, a perfectly oval face and a pair of cha-cha heels to carry it off.

➤ Soft side-swooped fringes suit girls with glasses – long hair with a fringe plus specs equals Cousin Itt from *The Addams Family.*

➤ Large Mekonesque fore- (or five) heads *always* need a fringe for camouflage, a fact that has bypassed Nicole Kidman. In 2008 a vitriolic Sharon Osbourne described Kidman's brow as a 'flat screen TV'.

➤ If you're thinking of a fringe, start off slowly – and long. Kate Moss's fringe is eye-skimming and broken up to look undone and suits her sun-kissed just-got-out-of-bed-with-the-latest-guitarist look.

➤ A chocolate coloured bob with a blunt-cut fringe is FIERCE and should be accompanied at all times with an Azzedine Alaia body con dress, opaque black Wolford tights and Manolo Blahnik cone heels.

➤ Never ever dry your fringe with a round brush – you'll look like Purdey as played by Joanna Lumley in *The New Avengers* circa 1976. Fine if you want to channel the 1970s but you're more likely to end up like Baldrick or Sean Ryder of the Happy Mondays circa 1988.

➤ Kate Moss does not use GHDs. Keep it fluffy.

❋ LEFT: Supermodel Kate Moss regularly has her hair cut with a choppy fringe before growing it out and starting all over again!

The Rules for Beautiful Hair
by Arlene Dahl

The quality of your hair, its suppleness and sheen, is of primary importance. The rules for beautiful hair are similar for those of a lovely complexion:

1 Keep it clean. It isn't true that frequent washing is bad for the hair. Stars working on movies usually have their hair washed every other day with no ill effects. So don't be afraid to wash your hair as often as necessary to keep it looking – and smelling – fresh.

2 Keep it stimulated – this is achieved by massaging the scalp and brushing the hair regularly. Massage your scalp after brushing. Place the fingertips on the scalp and massage with a circular motion, holding the fingers stationary but moving the scalp. Start with the hair that frames the face and gradually work around to the back and up to the crown. As you massage, you will feel the scalp becoming looser, so that it moves easily beneath your fingertips, relaxing its tightness and tension.

3 Keep it lubricated – hair that is dry and out of condition because of too much sun, a bad perm or a bad tinting job, can be restored with hot oil treatments, hair conditioners and cream hair masks.

4 Keep it scented – soft sweet-smelling hair makes men think of romance and springtime. Even in the dead of winter it's guaranteed to bring out the best (or the beast) in the male. Add a few drops of your favourite cologne to your rinse water after a shampoo, and rinse your combs and brushes in it, too.

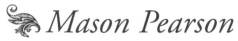# *Mason Pearson*
THE WORLD'S BEST HAIRBRUSH

Mason Pearson brushes are regarded as the Rolls Royce of hairbrushes. What makes them so special? Well, the most expensive in the Mason Pearson line, the All Boar Bristle has a rubber cushion in which is set all natural bristles. Unlike cheap nylon hairbrushes it untangles hair without damaging it, stimulates the scalp from root to tip and thus increases blood flow to the roots of the hair. Jean Kent described the ideal hairbrushing routine as follows:

1 Start at the ends of the hair and brush gently at first to remove any tangles, then gradually work up to the scalp.

2 Now brush the hair really vigorously, both sides and back, starting with the brush at the top of the head for each stroke.

3 Bend the head down and brush under the hair until you look like a Honolulu beauty.

4 Lastly, brush the hair down again.
These steps should be followed at least once a day.

The result – healthier, glossy hair. Kelly Brook, Catherine Zeta-Jones and Brooke Shields swear by its amazing results, as do hairdressers to the stars, including Ken Pave, who uses a Mason Pearson Junior Mixed Bristle on Jessica Simpson's golden locks. The world's best brush doesn't come cheap, however, prices can go up to $150 depending on the size. The upside is that if looked after properly it will literally last a lifetime so it's a one-time purchase. (mason-pearson.com or hqhair.com).

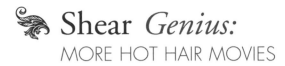

Shear *Genius:*
MORE HOT HAIR MOVIES

1928 PANDORA'S BOX (dir: G.W. Pabst) The definitive bob as worn by Louise Brooks.

1936 THE GARDEN OF ALLAH (dir: Richard Boleslawski) Watch Marlene Dietrich's hair in the oasis scenes – the wind blows the trees but her hair never ruffles!

1939 THE WOMEN (dir: George Cukor) A beautifully groomed Joan Crawford and Norma Shearer among a host of other 1930s glamourpusses. Many scenes are set in a Hollywood beauty salon – check out the perming machines!

1946 GILDA (dir: Charles Vidor) An iconic movie moment – Rita Hayworth tosses her hair as her introduction on screen. Born Margarita Carmen Cansino, Hollywood transformed a Spanish senorita into a red-headed Hayworth by lightening her jet-black hair and moving back her low hairline by one inch. It took three years of painful electrolysis to achieve the stunning results.

1953 ROMAN HOLIDAY (dir: William Wyler) Princess Ann played by Audrey Hepburn has a transformative haircut from long to short after she instructs the Italian barber, 'All off!' Many stars have tried but failed to get the same gamine look.

1958 VERTIGO (dir: Alfred Hitchcock) Kim Novak as a glacial blonde in a chignon and pencil skirt bewitches a bewildered James Stewart.

1960 À BOUT DE SOUFFLE (dir: Jean-Luc Godard) One of the most stylish and sexy movies ever made starring Jean-Paul Belmondo and Jean Seberg as star-crossed lovers in Left Bank Paris. Her close-cut crop is quite simply gorgeous.

1975 SHAMPOO (dir: Hal Ashby) Warren Beatty is a seriously seductive hairdressing super-stud who coifs an immaculate mid-length bob out of a chisel-cheeked Julie Christie.

1988 WORKING GIRL (dir: Mike Nichols) Textbook 1980s dress-for-success story in which Melanie Griffiths morphs from mall rat to executive chic as her perm and fringe combo is cut into a soft blonde bob.

Greer Garson's
Champagne Rinse

'IT'S AN *extravagance* THAT *shocks* MY SOUL, BUT I INDULGE ANYWAY! IT GIVES MY HAIR *body* AND *sparkle* AND MAKES ME FEEL *pampered* – LIKE CLEOPATRA DISSOLVING PEARLS IN VINEGAR.'

Shampoo your hair as normal, then rinse thoroughly with warm then cold water. For the final rinse, crack open the champers and pour over the head. Or, if you're feeling less flush, take half a cup of leftover flat champagne, mix with half a cup of hot water and use for the final rinse. DO NOT RINSE AGAIN! This luxe hair tip works particularly well on blondes to bring out the highlights.

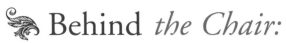 Behind *the Chair:*
WE REVEAL THE SECRETS OF THE STARS

➤ Actress CONSTANCE BENNETT used to shampoo her hair every two weeks with soap, then after rinsing rub in the whites of two eggs followed by several hot water rinses, then a tepid rinse, then plunge it into cold water.

➤ IRENE DUNNE had a hot oil rub three hours before shampooing, followed by a vinegar rinse – but only shampooed her hair once every three weeks!

➤ JUNE ALLYSON washed her hair twice a week in the shower massaging it vigorously through three shampoos, then thoroughly rinsed it and then set it in curlers with beer.

➤ THE DUCHESS OF WINDSOR (A.K.A. MRS SIMPSON) used to have her hair dressed three times a day; in the morning to go under a little hat, in the afternoon to go to the races and in the evening with a hair ornament. Each hairdo took half an hour. She used a special shampoo made of five egg yolks and two measures of rum.

➤ MARILYN MONROE used Wella Kolestral Concentrate, a conditioning crème. You can still buy it today from hairproducts.com.

➤ When EVA LONGORIA needs a quick root touch-up her hairdresser spritzes them with hairspray and then uses eyeshadow the same colour as her hair dye to blend them in.

➤ MADONNA intentionally lets her roots show through – it gives an edgy undone look to pristine blonde hair. But she's over 50 so why aren't they grey?

➤ JENNIFER LOPEZ rinses her hair in mineral water – it flattens the hair cuticles and boosts the shine.

➤ A tip from DANIEL GALVIN – if you are colouring your hair at home and get it on your hairline mix up cigarette ash with a little water and rub gently at the stain. It will come away easily!

➤ SOPHIA LOREN cuts her own fringe.

➤ JERRY HALL only washes her hair once a week and NEVER blow-dries it. She uses French mink oil on the ends and brushes with a trusty Mason Pearson.

'I CAN'T GET BY WITHOUT MY
48 Hairbrush BY MASON PEARSON.
Kate Moss WON'T LEAVE HOME
WITHOUT HERS.'

James Brown on Kate Moss

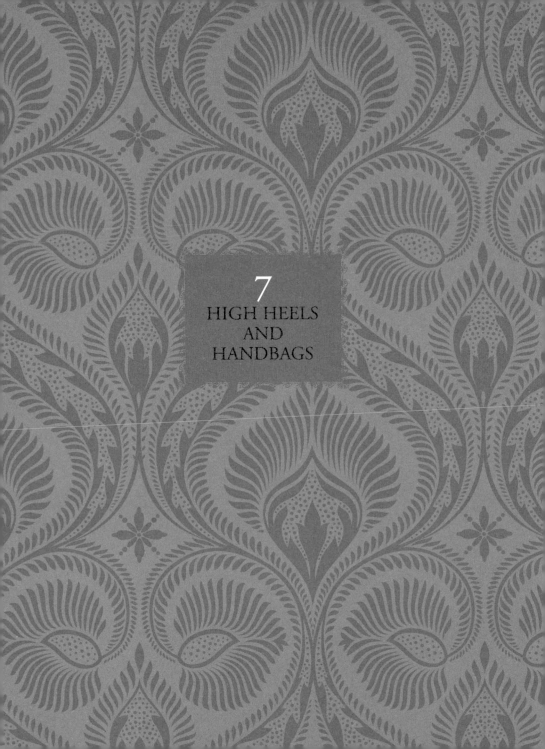

7
HIGH HEELS
AND
HANDBAGS

HIGH HEELS
AND HANDBAGS

Joan Crawford could be speaking for many of us when she commented, 'bags and shoes are my weakness.' In her day a girl wouldn't leave the house until she was perfectly put together with a matching bag and heels, a hat, gloves and costume jewellery. Accessorizing was an art passed down from mother to daughter with advice gleaned from fan magazines and beauty books. Today accessories have never been more fashion forward but we seem to have lost the glamourpuss art of wearing them with élan.

The glamourpuss of the past knew that a sassy pair of heels and a cute crocodile clutch could lift an ordinary outfit into fashion's stratosphere and create a frisson of anticipation in any red blooded male and a round of applause from her girlfriends. Marilyn Monroe, Audrey Hepburn and Doris Day knew that the right accessory marked a girl out from the crowd as someone with style, sex appeal and exquisite taste. So in Doris Day's words, 'Why not gild the lily? Why not use accessories, jewellery, perfume – anything to help make you more attractive to the opposite sex?' Indulging your fashion fantasies is also an adorable way to bond with other like-minded women who appreciate the more subtle nuances of glamourpuss style and will enthusiastically egg you on in the pursuit of high heels, handbags, baubles and beads. What (heterosexual) man would ever do that!

Marilyn Monroe's
Shoe Secrets

* Always wear flesh-coloured shoes with flesh-coloured stockings, black with black and always, always high heels because they lengthen the legs. A different coloured stocking to the heel breaks up the line and makes your leg look shorter. Marilyn commissioned her favourite shoe designers to make special flesh-toned silk shoes to match her stockings.

* Follow the same rules at night but make sure the heels are encrusted with rhinestones!

* Find a shoe designer whose styles work for you and stick with him or her. Marilyn had 40 pairs of Ferragamos.

Hooray *for High Heels!*

Many of us would rather take a trip to hell in high heels than walk flat-heeled into heaven – we know that a good pair of heels is every woman's best friend. They not only add instant glamour, but also erotic allure by lengthening the legs, arching the back and forcing the tush and chest up … and out. Meow!!

They can also boost your sex life, according to Dr Maria Cerruto, who hit the headlines in 2008 when she found that the altered posture given by regularly wearing a 5cm (2") and higher heel improved the pelvic muscles and their ability to contract – leading to more and better orgasms! No wonder men and women find a high heel sexy and none more so than Marilyn Monroe, who said they 'gave a lift to her career'.

Every star has her must-have designer shoe. For Marilyn Monroe it was Salvatore Ferragamo, an Italian label that still dominates the European luxury market. She had 40 pairs ranging from satin tapered heels by day and gold kidskin at night. Audrey Hepburn also had a penchant for Ferragamo's black leather court shoes as an alternative to her ubiquitous ballet flats. Today the name on every celebrity's lips is Christian Louboutin, whose shoes are on the feet of Victoria Beckham, Angelina Jolie, Kylie Minogue and Gwyneth Paltrow. Sarah Jessica Parker's passion for Manolo Blahnik's creations is well known – she admits to owning more than a hundred pairs. Like the stars of the past Parker is happy to suffer for her heels and is honest about the condition of her feet, saying, 'I've destroyed my feet completely, but I don't care. What do you really need your feet for anyway?'

At least she's honest, high heels are never going to be more comfortable than flip-flops and most major stars like Parker have a limo round the corner waiting for them after a five minute meet-and-greet. The rest of us aren't so lucky. It takes a lot of practice to move in high heels and even longer to develop what supermodel Tyra Banks calls a 'signature walk'. Way before, Marilyn Monroe realized that a wiggly walk could be her calling card, a walk that comedian Groucho Marx said 'made smoke come out of my head'.

Every time Marilyn took a step, she wobbled on her ankles causing a corresponding tremor through her derrière and breasts. Speculation was rife over what made her do this – explanations included a swimming accident, double-jointed knees and a fractured foot as a child, all of which she denied saying:

> 'I'VE *never* DONE ANYTHING DELIBERATELY ABOUT THE *way I walk*. PEOPLE SAY I WALK ALL *wiggly* AND *wobbly*, BUT I DON'T KNOW WHAT THEY MEAN. I JUST *walk*. I'VE *never* WRIGGLED DELIBERATELY IN MY LIFE.'

She was not prepared to give away her secret but Jimmy Starr, former columnist on the *Los Angeles Herald Express*, was: 'She learned a trick of cutting a quarter of an inch off one heel so that when she walked her little fanny would wriggle.'

The Stiletto's Sex Appeal

The most extreme version of the high heel is the stiletto –
the Hollywood heel favoured by the sexiest of old school
stars and present day bombshells – Jayne Mansfield had
200 pairs. Let's face it, they are pretty tough on the feet
(some of us have the bunions to prove it) but the pay-off is
increased height and a kind of super-femininity. At 10–12cm
(4–5") and above, stilettos are still a high fashion must-have
today and remain shoes of status, authority and sex appeal.
The sexiest killer heels are those by Christian Louboutin,
whose covetable Very Prive and Bruges stilettos are some
of the highest in the business.

Louboutin's stilettos are instantly recognizable because they have bright
red soles. The idea came while the designer was working on a collection
that was influenced by the American Pop artist Andy Warhol. After the
initial design drawings were done, Louboutin felt something was
missing and noticed that one of the assistants was painting her nails in
bright red lacquer. He took the bottle and painted the soles of the
shoes with the gloss so that though some of the shoes looked demure
on the outside, once a woman was walking they gave a flirtatious flash.
This is the only form of advertising Louboutin has ever done, and it's
subliminal, subversive and sexy like the shoes themselves.

Banish Cankles by Jean Kent

*When there is no discernible narrowing between calf, ankle
and foot you have cankles (calf + ankle = cankle).*

'A slim, graceful ankle is a thing of beauty
and many a woman has a pretty ankle to
thank for her claim to beauty. If, however,
you think your ankles are a little too plump,
do not despair, here are a few remedies:

➤ 'When sitting reading a book, or
mending, gently rotate each foot. Another
exercise that can be done in bed is to
stretch each foot in turn with the toe
pointing downwards and rotate the foot.
This exercise should be done for ten
minutes night and morning.

➤ 'Remove your slippers, raise yourself as
high as you can on your toes and, keeping
your legs as stiff as possible, walk about the
room taking tiny Chinese steps. This exercise
need not interfere with your movements
e.g. journeys to the wardrobe and back to
the dressing table, or longer ones to the
bathroom, can all be made while you are
beautifying your ankles.'

Audrey Hepburn's *Ballet Flats*

The right shoe can conjure up a fashion moment of pure unalloyed glamour: Terry de Havilland's towering wedges in pastel and gold python skin summon the spirit of Bianca Jagger or Jerry Hall strutting their stuff in a strobe lit 1970s discotheque; the ballet flat means the ever-elegant Audrey Hepburn in a black crew-necked sweater and cropped Capri pants moving to cool jazz in a smoky Left Bank drinking den.

Audrey's flats were by Salvatore Ferragamo, who made her a pair in black suede with a low oval heel and shell sole. She also shopped for ballet flats at Capezio, a New York firm specializing in dance wear that has been in existence for more than a hundred years. Capezio still produce the 1950s ballet flats that Audrey wore and they can be bought online at capeziodance.com. The same style, but especially designed to be more hard-wearing for pounding the pavements of city streets are those by French Sole a company that started in 1989 as a concept company that sold only ballet-style footwear. Style is the operative word for this company who produce ballet flats that have the look of the original dancing shoe but with more functional hard-wearing soles. Their Lowcut and Henrietta styles are worn by Kate Moss and Sienna Miller and are a sure-fire way of getting the Audrey look, but in a much more modern and practical way. And Audrey's tip? 'Always buy a pair of shoes half a size bigger, as comfort is integral to elegance.'

❋ RIGHT: Audrey Hepburn dressed in the understated Beatnik style of the 1950s. Her classic black wool crewneck, Capri pants and ballet flats remain a uniform of cool.

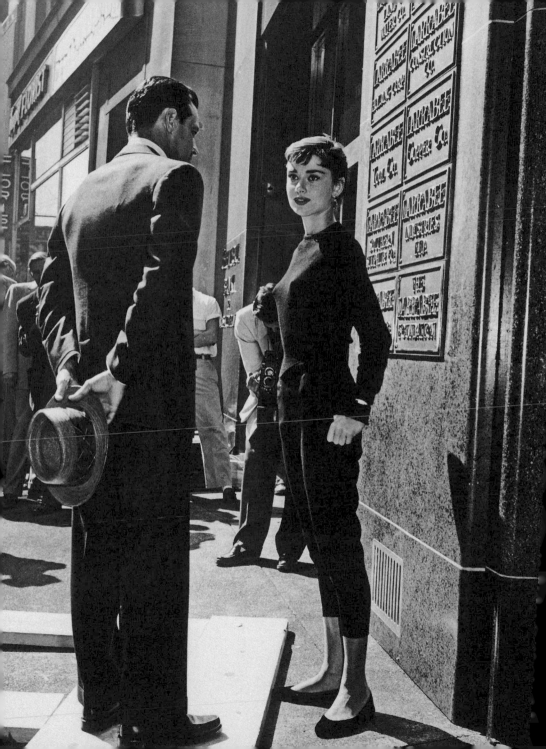

The Handbag

A woman's handbag is almost an extension of her body. There are few swains man enough to let their fingertips roam a bag's dark velvety depths. The freedom we modern women enjoy means that we have more places to be, more people to see and more and more fabulously designed handbags to buy.

Some stars' handbags are instantly recognizable – the Hermès Kelly, for instance, as sported by Victoria Beckham in a variety of colours to match each outfit. This covetable *objet de luxe* was named after the effortlessly elegant Grace Kelly was snapped by paparazzi while attempting to conceal her pregnancy with one in 1956. As only 60 are made each season, it's also one of the world's most expensive starting at $4,000 for the most basic model. Jackie O is most usually associated with the Gucci 0633, a miniature bag in beige calf with a bamboo handle, and when she wore the Gucci Constance shoulderbag in the 1960s so many women asked for 'Jackie's bag with the double strap and H clasp' that Gucci renamed it the Jackie O.

In the 1920s silent movie star Mary Pickford carried a gold and black enamel clutch by Cartier that had a tiny tube of lipstick built inside. Every time it ran out, it had to be sent back to the jewellers to be refilled. Madonna started her own It Bag craze in the 1990s with her selection of Fendi Baguettes in apple-green sequins, zebra stripe and hot pink snakeskin. Princess Diana consistently carried the Lady Dior in black crocodile with gold charms that spelled out the Dior logo. This Sloane Ranger Special has been referred to as the leather equivalent of a yapping chihuahua.

5 KEY HANDBAG SHAPES

BAGUETTE A bag with a short strap and worn tucked under the arm. Named after the French loaf of bread that has a similar (if longer) shape.

CLUTCH Invented in the 1920s, can snap shut in the middle or have an envelope flap. Called a clutch because it's clutched or gripped under the upper arm or in the hand. Pretty impractical for everyday, as one arm or hand is put out of use; clutches can also be really easily lost or forgotten.

HOBO An oversized soft leather bag in a curved crescent shape with a shoulder strap. First fashionable in the 1970s when designed in expensive grades of buttery leather by Carlos Falchi. Named after the traditional image of a hobo or tramp carrying his belongings hanging off the end of a stick.

TOTE A large flat bag with an open top and zippered pockets inside. Traditionally used to 'tote' around while shopping but in deluxe materials can be elevated to must-have status. Mulberry's super-sized Roxanne Tote in navy vinyl will set you back $1,000!

MINAUDIÈRE A rigid evening clutch that traditionally combined a purse and an evening bag. First appeared in the 1930s after Charles Arpel of jewellers Van Cleef & Arpels saw socialite Florence Gould carrying her make-up and cigarette lighter in a tin usually reserved for Lucky Strike cigarettes. The first minaudières were intricately engineered metal boxes with lots of hidden compartments. The name derives from the French 'minauder', which means 'to simper', a habit for which Van Cleef's wife, Estelle, was notorious!

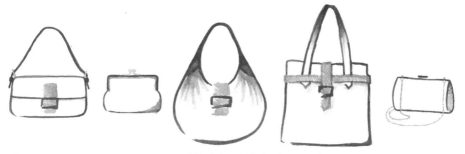

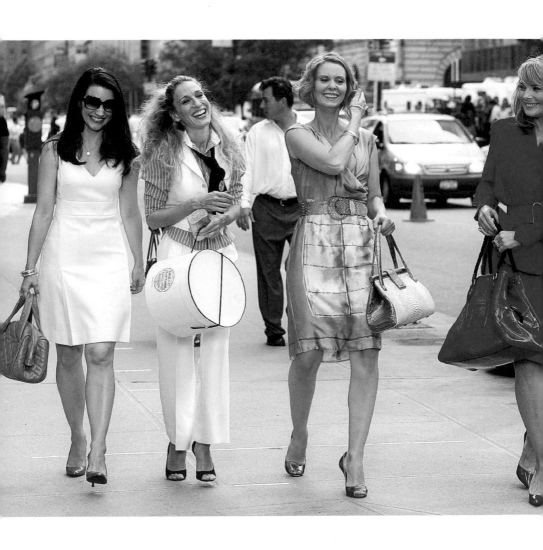

✳ ABOVE: The *Sex and The City* cast turned New York's sidewalks into global catwalks. They helped kick-start the 2000s obsession with accessories.

🌿 Bags *of Personality*

Take four fashionistas – Carrie, Miranda, Charlotte and Samantha of *Sex and The City* fame. Each with their own distinct personality and accessories to match, courtesy of über stylist Patricia Field. You've avidly consumed their images on the TV and movie screen and been transported to a glamorous fashion heaven full of gladiator heels and outlandish corsages. Now it's time for you to decide if you have the persona to fit right in should you alight at JFK. Are you a sexy Samantha or a quirky Carrie, a classic Charlotte or careerist Miranda? And most importantly – do you have the bag to match? (From left to right)

CHARLOTTE

A Fifth Avenue traditionalist with a blithely peppy personality. At home in classic, discreetly expensive styles such as this simple white shift accessorized with a Chanel double C logoed bowler in beige quilted lambskin retailing at over $3,000. If you dream of a Kennedy blond knight in shining armour to sweep you off your feet and can find your way around the place settings in the most top-notch of restaurants, this is your bag. Look for quilted leather, introduced into bag design by Coco Chanel in her 1955 classic the 2.55. This black leather shoulderbag was named after its month and year of birth. The Chanel style is all understatement; chic creams, black,

navy and beige combined with gilt hardware that accents simple silhouettes. It's a look that has been endlessly copied on the high street since the 1960s so look in your local thrift stores and flea markets as well as classic retailers such as Marks & Spencer and other leading department stores.

CARRIE

The city fashionista is a quirky catwalk flirt who openly questions relationships but believes in the power of old fashioned romance. If you're a fashion leader rather than fashion follower, anticipating trends before they hit the high street and openly challenging fashion's status quo, Carrie's eccentric arm candy is for you. In the movie her bags include a Timmy Woods Eiffel Tower bag encrusted in Swarovski crystals, Salvatore Ferragamo's Pheasant Feather bag and here a tiny yet deluxe Judith Leiber Wavy Curve Ombre Clutch with a snap flap and hidden chain strap alongside a huge hat box. Leiber's tiny minaudières are sleek metal boxes of considerable beauty and intricate craftsmanship – so very expensive! To get the Carrie look, go for unusual feather/material/leather combinations and Surrealist shapes that disguise the handbags' function. Don't be afraid to mix a floral dress with a feather bag, stripes with spots or matte and patent leathers in jewel bright hues.

MIRANDA

A career-driven lawyer who juggles the demands of home, work and play, becoming a little cynical as a result. If your friends see you as the voice of reason and you're equally at home in both boardroom and bedroom you will relate to Miranda's flawlessly fitted and polished style. In this scene her bag is the most deluxe, a stratospherically expensive Nancy Gonzalez Frame handbag in python and crocodile skin designed by the self styled Queen

of Croc in her native Colombia. Gonzalez's bags are some of the most expensive in the world, identifiable because of their expanses of flawless skin with little visible hardware to break up the lines. The simple reptile bag dominated the 1950s and literally thousands were produced. You can pick up a really inexpensive one on ebay or in a vintage store at a fraction of the price of a modern bag, and the original unfarmed skin will undoubtedly be of much higher quality than its modern equivalent.

SAMANTHA

A pure fashion powerhouse who channels 1980s status dressing by wearing bright brash colours and body hugging silhouettes. If you're an extrovert who loves all eyes upon you as you sashay down the city streets, and you take no prisoners when it comes to the men in your life, this over-sized Fendi du Jour bag is for you. It's shiny, sexy and sassy in bright red patent leather, laser cut with polka dots and logo star-shaped studs. You won't get the design detail cheaply but a full-on Samantha vibe can be created by wearing one pure primary colour, like this pillar box red with a matching tote in PVC.

How to Spot a
Fake Bag at Fifty Paces

❧ It's all about quality! Fake Hermès are really easy to spot as the real deal is handmade from start to finish and has more than 2,600 hand stitches, a flap closure with a gold buckle and four tiny gold feet on which the bag stands to stop the bottom wearing out.

❧ Check the bag has an authenticity card and serial number. If still in doubt, ask to see the original receipt.

❧ Look at the hardware. Many high end designer bags have embossed logos on the sides of buckles and links on chain straps to make them harder to counterfeit.

❧ Patterns like the monogram on Louis Vuitton bags are always perfectly symmetrical. Any asymmetry instantly denotes a fake.

Elizabeth *Taylor:*
BIG GIRLS WEAR BIG DIAMONDS

Elizabeth Taylor has a lust for diamonds that almost matches her lust for male flesh and Kate Moss follows suit today with her own vast collection of vintage rocks. In 1968 actor Richard Burton, the most infamous of Liz's many mates, paid $305,000 for the Krupp diamond, 33.19 carats of flawless ice that his wife was renowned for leaving by the sink in the ladies' powder room after removing it to wash her hands. This fabulous diamond was followed closely by the Cartier (re-named Taylor-Burton) at 69.42 carats and a cool $1.1m.

We can't all afford rocks as big as The Ritz but there is one classic genre of jewellery that is within the reach of most girls' purses – pearls. A simple pair of pearl studs plus matching necklace immediately evoke the classic American understatement of Grace Kelly. The traditional way to buy a pearl necklace is by length; a collar, as worn by Grace, sits at the base of the neck and measures 25–33cm (10–13"); a princess length hangs just below the collarbone and is 43–48cm (17–19"); a matinée falls just above the décolleté at 50–60cm (20–24"); and an opera is longer at 70–90cm (28–35"). The longest length of pearls is called a rope and comes in at any measurement longer than the opera – this flapper-style pearl necklace was worn by Louise Brooks in the 1920s.

In 1969 Richard Burton bought one of the world's largest black pearls La Peregrina, which originally belonged to King Philip II of Spain. Soon after he presented it to Elizabeth Taylor, she lost it. She resonantly describes her panic in her book, *My Love Affair with Jewelry.*

'I WENT OUT AND SORT OF STARTED HUMMING "*lalala*", AND I WAS WALKING BACK AND FORTH IN MY BARE FEET, SEEING IF I WOULD FIND ANYTHING IN THE CARPET. I WAS TRYING TO BE COMPOSED AND LOOK AS IF I HAD A PURPOSE BECAUSE INSIDE I WAS PRACTICALLY HEAVING, I WAS *so upset*. I LOOKED OVER AND SAW THE WHITE PEKINGESE … AND I SAW ONE CHEWING ON A BONE. AND I DID THE *longest, slowest* DOUBLE TAKE IN MY HEAD. I JUST CASUALLY OPENED THE PUPPY'S MOUTH AND INSIDE HIS MOUTH WAS THE MOST *perfect pearl* IN THE WORLD. IT WAS – *thank God* – NOT SCRATCHED. I DID FINALLY TELL RICHARD. BUT I HAD TO WAIT *at least* A WEEK!'

Elizabeth Taylor

Eight Jewellery Tips
by Doris Day

➤ Earrings add piquancy to any kind
of dress whether silk, satin, cotton
or denim.

➤ For an after dark date, a pair of pearl stud
earrings and matching choker is the
perfect combination. If you're wearing
black it's unbeatable.

➤ Fake jewellery is fine as long as it's not
too conspicuous.

➤ Wear four to five delicate gold bangles
on one wrist.

➤ Wrap an old fashioned locket around
one wrist.

➤ A set of diamond earrings will make you
feel like a million dollars – fake or not!

➤ You don't have to be rich to be chic!

➤ Good taste is easily developed.

Boys Do Make Passes at Girls Who Wear Glasses
by Petula Clark

'Dorothy Parker could not have been more wrong when she made that by now famous remark about gents not making passes at girls who wear glasses. Despite the spectacles on my nose I've never had any trouble getting dates. My spectacles certainly never worried any of my boyfriends!

'I wear glasses almost everywhere, except when I'm acting on the set or taking a shower! And I've never been a wallflower at parties or dances. I've heard as many wolf-calls as most girls, specs or no specs!

'Why hide them when you've got to wear them? That's impractical vanity, and only leads to a near-sighted girl smacking her nose against a door because she can't see where she's going. Glasses can improve your appearance. They can appear to shorten your nose. Or they can make your face look narrow or wide according to the shape of the frame! Even if they make you look the "intellectual type" – is that bad?'

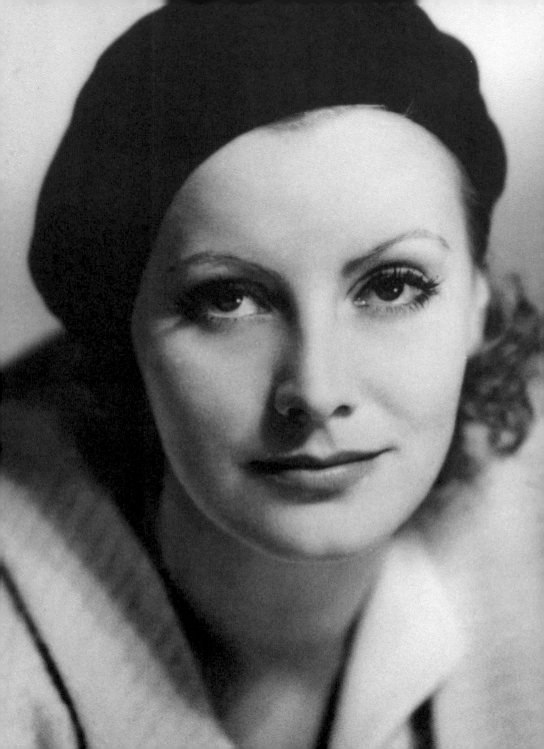

How to Wear a Beret
Like Greta Garbo

In the movie *The Gay Deception* of 1935 an elderly man is giving advice: 'Young man, I'll tell you a secret – just between men. All women's hats are monstrosities. That's a secret we men must carry to our graves.'

OK so hats are difficult. You're only one small step away from an up-turned bucket or looking like a cheap version of Boy George in a off centre titfer by Stephen Jones. But the beret is different especially when worn by Garbo. In films Garbo's beret can be a little over-styled but once off the film set she wore a beret with natural aplomb. The trick is to pull it right down so it covers the entire head and then push it back so it lies just above the hairline – this prevents the flying saucer effect. The best authentic Basque berets are by Borsalino and Elosegui made out of felted wool and dyed black or navy blue. Look out for a strip of leather stitched inside the headband – this makes the beret fit more securely. Go to any store that stocks Kangol for a less structured example in angora. Check out berets.com for anything beret related.

LEFT: The ubiquitous Greta Garbo shows how to wear a beret – once you get it right mix with a classic trench and a pair of correspondent shoes for an instant air of MI5!

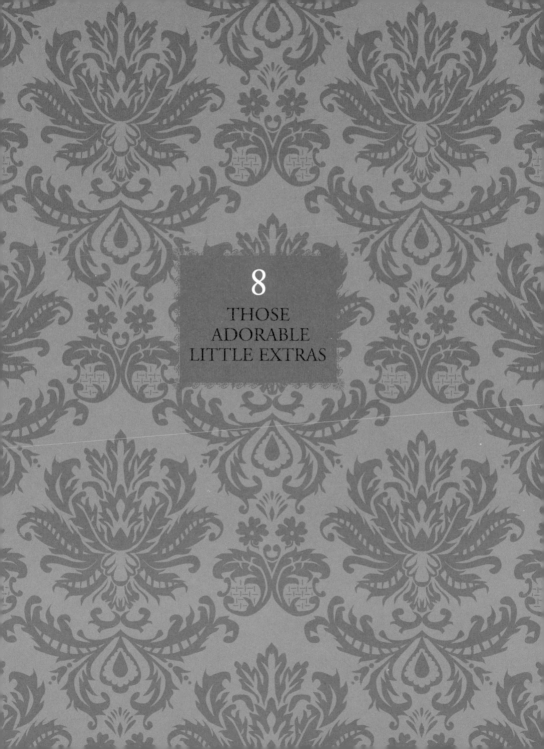

8
THOSE
ADORABLE
LITTLE EXTRAS

THOSE ADORABLE LITTLE EXTRAS

Being truly adorable means eschewing the more vulgar trappings of superstardom. Angelina Jolie doesn't flaunt her wealth by living as luxuriously as the reigning dynasties of Europe. Solid gold bathtubs and Beluga caviar are not Reese Witherspoon's style. Carla Bruni doesn't swank around in sable and sapphires – discreet dove grey Dior is the order of her day. Truly adorable women don't need their latest beau to festoon them with magnolia blossoms and have no use for Jacobean crewel curtains, a private island or an Afghan hound. They are adored because of their dramatic physical presence, their exquisite poses and peppy personality, their graceful body language – and the traces of history they leave in some very special places.

Just think what a weight would be taken off your mind if you were to start your own seismic shift in the frenetic world of fashion. By refusing to participate in bin-end bargain hunting in a feeble attempt to ape the latest vapid catwalk looks, you would have time to take a deep breath, step back and look at the bigger picture. Adorable little extras like a vintage Burberry trench, a pearl buttoned cashmere cardigan and a winning smile can last a lifetime, and if accessorized with an elegant pose, a whimsical pet and a lurid cocktail in an appropriate setting, heaven knows what might ensue?

'I *love* LUXURY. AND LUXURY LIES NOT IN RICHNESS AND ORNATENESS BUT IN THE ABSENCE OF *vulgarity*. VULGARITY IS THE *ugliest* WORD IN OUR LANGUAGE. I STAY IN THE GAME TO *fight* IT.'

Coco Chanel

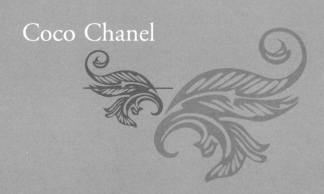

🌿 *Making an Entrance*

For those around you to think that *you have got it all going on*, you need to fake it a little. The best way to do this is to make a dramatic entrance – even if it's all downhill from there on in, people will still continue to reverberate with your illustrious presence! In 1962 Elizabeth Taylor glided onto the set of *Cleopatra* in a floor-skimming black mink coat followed by a retinue that included two hairdressers and costume designers, a secretary, maid and press agent. It was the first day of shooting. She walked past her co-stars Rex Harrison and Richard Burton with imperious ease and stopped in front of the director Joseph L. Mankiewicz.

> 'Are you ready, my Queen?' he enquired, as he took her small, plump hand and kissed it.
> 'I was born ready, dear Sir,' she replied as she dropped her mink to the floor to reveal a dazzling skin-tight gold beaded gown.
> 'My dear, you leave me breathless,' swooned Jo.
> 'Of course I do,' she replied.

Joan Crawford's entrances were equally impressive. In 1929 she became one half of a celebrated Hollywood power couple when she married Douglas Fairbanks Junior, despite his parents' disapproval – not least because she was rumoured to have played a starring role in quite a few stag movies on her rise to the top. Douglas's mother, Mary Pickford, sniffed with disdain whenever Joan was mentioned and referred to her new daughter-in-law as her son's current chorus girl fling. Three months after the wedding the bride and her in-laws had yet to meet and this was causing a few negative headlines in the Hollywood press. Mary grudgingly invited Joan to a sumptuous dinner party in honour of Lord and Lady Mountbatten held at Pickfair, her fabulous home in the Hollywood Hills. Timing her arrival to the millisecond, Joan turned up in full battle-gear, namely an ornate white lace dress with a matching bag and white lace heels. As she entered the foyer, she saw that all the esteemed guests were mingling on the floor below. The butler took her white fur wrap and as Joan approached the steps and saw her father-in-law approaching to greet her, she stopped and posed at the top.

'Wait!' she hissed to her husband out of the corner of her mouth, 'I think the strap of my shoe's come undone!'
'Welcome to Pickfair, Joan' said Douglas Senior.
'My shoe, it's undone!' whispered Joan in distress!
Both Douglas' Junior and Senior bent down simultaneously to fasten it. With both men literally kneeling at her feet, Joan's eyes swept the crowd, sought out the steely glare of Mary Pickford. She smiled ever so sweetly back.

First things first – get your posture right so you can make the most dramatic of entrances. Not every girl is born beautiful but every girl can carry herself as if she were! You may have some bad habits ingrained over the years but it's well worth sorting them out. Inexpensive clothes worn with the right air can look a million dollars, while fashion's latest duds, if worn with an apologetic droop, lose a lot of their glamour.

How to Walk Tall

1950s fashion journalist and advisor to the stars Constance Moore said, 'Good posture is easy posture. If you watch someone who is really graceful, you will see that they seem relaxed and effortless.' Here are her tips for perfect posture:

➤ Begin your attempts towards improved deportment with a deliberate relaxing of all muscle tension. Relaxing is not the same thing as flopping. You can sit or stand upright, yet be free from tension.

➤ Stand squarely with your feet together, arms by your sides: if you stand quite naturally your thumbs should come an inch or two in front of your side skirt seams.

➤ Get your head as high as possible, not by raising the chin but by imagining your two ears are being drawn upwards by a magnet. Balancing a book on your head will give you the right head position.

➤ Now draw the muscles of your waist and tummy upwards and slightly in. In other words, stand tall; but relax, don't stand stiffly.

➤ From this position take three slow, even breaths, then drop forward, allowing your arms and head to hang loosely down to the floor. Your back should be relaxed and rounded. Hold this position for three more slow breaths, stretching downwards a little on each. Then come back up to the starting position and repeat the whole movement three times.

➤ Having achieved the correct standing position, try to maintain it while walking or sitting.

※ RIGHT: Diana's posture reflected her increasing confidence. Her once bashful stoop was replaced by a straight backed elegance as she realized the benefit of walking tall.

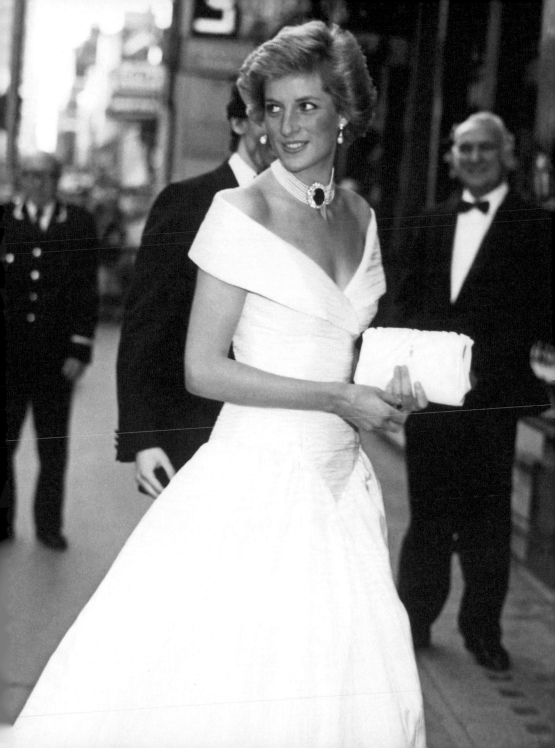

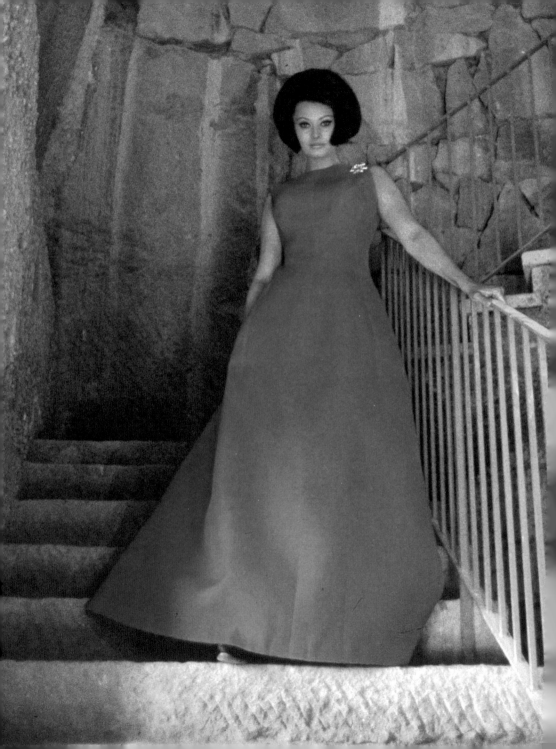

How to Descend a Staircase
Movie-Star-Style

Pause at the top and look around for a
few seconds – people will immediately gaze
at you trying to determine who you are.
Check discreetly for any small dogs, toys
or skateboards lying around and start
descending. If you're wearing a long skirt
hold up the hem with your free hand so it
doesn't get caught under your heels whilst
delicately running your hand along the rail
with the other, ready to grip if things get
dicey. Do not, under any circumstances look
at your feet. Keep your head up and smile –
or like showgirl Mistinguett paint fake eyes
on your eyelids so that when you're looking
down it looks as if you're looking ahead!

✳ LEFT: Sophia Loren descends a staircase in perfect
glamourpuss style – eyes front, head erect and skirt
discreetly held so as not to hamper her movements.

How to Pose for a Photograph
Like Victoria Beckham

Maybe you haven't noticed, but Victoria Beckham poses in a very particular way at press launches and red carpet events. She puts her hands at back of her waist and pushes her torso slightly backwards and her shoulders forwards so the centre of her body curves inwards. This creates a concave that draws attention to her tiny waist and flat belly. It's copied from the poses struck by models such as Dorian Leigh and Suzy Parker at 1950s couture shows and *Vogue* photoshoots – John Galliano gets his models to do it today. It gives instant class and elegance and gets away from the cheesy one-hand-on-hip stance that many stars automatically adopt.

Adorable Hotels

Once you've mastered the art of being the most perfectly adorable guest in your local area, it's time to take your wondrousness abroad! You may not be able to rent a room in the following sumptuous surroundings but you can always order coffee! The trick is to find out what's available to non-residents – most hotels have a bar or coffee shop that you can use, even a lobby where you can pose and have your photo taken! Book a cheap flight and a motel room then swan into the swankier parts of town looking adorable.

1 THE BEVERLY HILLS HOTEL, LOS ANGELES

Gloria Swanson stayed here, the divine Garbo hid here and Katharine Hepburn jumped fully clothed into the pool after a strenuous game of tennis. The Beverly Hills Hotel in Los Angeles remains the enclave of the chosen few including Cindy Crawford, Jessica Alba, Mariah Carey and Katie Holmes. This iconic pink stucco building (a.k.a. The Pink Palace) with its discreet bungalows scattered around the grounds has seen all sorts of salacious activity since its doors opened in 1912 – Carole Lombard and Clark Gable made mad passionate love in No. 5 while waiting for his divorce to come through, and Marilyn Monroe and Yves Montand chose the hotel for their short-lived affair. Marilyn, in fact, had quite a penchant for the Beverly Hills Hotel. In 1952, after her lease had run out in a house in the Hollywood Hills, she moved into a room on the third floor. At Christmas, returning from a studio party expecting to spend the night alone, she opened the door to find a twinkling Christmas tree, a blazing log fire and champagne on ice courtesy of her boyfriend (later husband) baseball star Joe DiMaggio. She often referred to it as her 'best Christmas ever'.

Eccentric billionaire Howard Hughes rented three bungalows throughout the 1950s whether he used them or not. One was for his wife, one for himself and one for his bodyguards – it cost more than $2 million dollars a year. Such was his obsession with privacy that the roast beef sandwiches he ordered from room service had to be left in a special fork in a tree in the garden so he could retrieve and eat them in private, a prelude to his last days as a germ-obsessed recluse.

Now staying here is expensive, $275 a night *at least* and it also has a snooty card referencing system – white for civilians, blue for the regular rich and pink for superstars. But you can come in as a non-resident to eat and soak up the atmosphere at The Polo Lounge – the famous eatery from which Mia Farrow was banned in the 1960s for wearing trousers. There's also the Cabana Club Café, where you can pose poolside, the Tea Lounge that has a gold baby grand piano, and cheapest of all the Fountain Coffee Shop, where you can get an inexpensive American breakfast or a toasted sandwich and strawberry milkshake. The ambience is enhanced by the original 1949 curved counter surrounded by wallpaper emblazoned with banana leaves and a working soda fountain.
The Beverly Hills Hotel, 9641 Sunset Boulevard, Beverly Hills, USA
thebeverlyhillshotel.com

2 COPACABANA PALACE
HOTEL, RIO DE JANEIRO

Brazil means glamourpuss Carmen Miranda, she of the tutti-frutti hat, polka dot ruffles and magnificent sequin-encrusted wedges. It's also where you can find, after flying down to Rio, this fabulous Art Deco hotel built in 1923. This is where Dolores del Rio broke up with boyfriend Orson Welles – so incensed was he that he threw all the furniture into the swimming pool. Ava Gardner fled here after breaking up with Frank Sinatra, Jayne Mansfield caused a scandal by sunbathing topless and swashbuckling actor Erroll Flynn ran naked through the hallways. Princess Diana and Marlene Dietrich have stayed – Marlene is said to have worn a dress so tight for a performance here she requested a bucket of sand in her dressing room for use as a temporary loo because she couldn't walk to the ladies.

While the rooms are out of bounds to most of us, sipping a caipirinha in the Piano Bar or at the poolside Pérgula Restaurant isn't. Enjoy half a dozen oysters or a lacquered duck thigh while imagining Orson's trouser press plummeting in with a splash. Then get up, go round the corner and visit the Carmen Miranda Museum at the Avenue Rui Barbosa Flamengo – as small and adorable as her!
Copacabana Palace, Avenue Atlântica 1702, Rio de Janeiro, Brazil
copacabanapalace.com.br

3 PARCO DEI PRINCIPI, SORRENTO

Perched on a clifftop overlooking the bright blue Gulf of Naples this is the place to pose in a Pucci shift and a pair of Ferragamos. Italy was the destination of choice in the late 1950s and early 1960s and you can live *la dolce vita* (if only for an afternoon) at this hotel. It's an astonishing time capsule of Italian postwar style by the genius of Italian designer Gio Ponti. Walk through the wrought iron gates off a dusty road of budget hotels and you will immediately start channelling Gina Lollobrigida as you walk through lush gardens with towering palm trees, two startlingly sculptural swimming pools and then the stark white modernism of the hotel building. Take a deep breath, hold your head high and walk into the lobby. Turn right and you're in the bright blue and white bar. Here you can perch on Ponti chairs, all blue vinyl with typically 1960s splayed wooden legs and look at the totally untouched interior complete with the same tiles, lampshades and furniture that were put there by Ponti in 1962. *Belissimo!*
Parco dei Principi, Via Rota 1, Sorrento, Italy
grandhotelparcodeiprincipi.net

4 LE CARLTON, CANNES

The Carlton opened in 1911, its design which incorporates two large cupolas is said to have been modelled on the breasts on one of France's most famous courtesans, La Belle Otero, who famously said, 'no man who has an account at Cartier's can be regarded as ugly.' Otero was a Spanish dancer described in the French press as 'the most scandalous person since Helen of Troy'. Men found her absolutely irresistible – a fact of which she was only too aware, saying, 'Ever since my childhood, I have been accustomed to see the face of every man who passed me light with desire. Is it so despicable to be the flower whose perfume people long to inhale, the fruit they long to taste?' Her list of lovers spanned Europe and included the Prince of Wales (who gave her a hunting lodge outside Paris where they could meet for a little tryst now and then), King Alfonso XIII of Spain and Nicholas, Czar of Russia. At the Carlton La Belle Otero could be spotted stalking to her special table, her face powdered and rouged, her eyes rimmed with kohl, trailing chinchilla and clouds of ylang-ylang, her latest lover in tow. After a life of dissolution, Otero died unrepentant at the age of 97.

Some of the world's most famous couples have stayed here – Prince Aly Khan and Rita Hayworth honeymooned at the Carlton in 1949, closely followed by Elizabeth Taylor and her first husband Nicky Hilton in 1950. Grace Kelly and Prince Rainier of Monaco met for a photo shoot at the hotel during the 1955 Cannes Film Festival, where she was publicizing Hitchcock's *To Catch a Thief* in which she starred with Cary Grant. And on that note, before hanging out there you MUST watch the movie as it uses the Carlton as its central location and it plays a pivotal role in the plot. Grace and Cary have several scenes on the private beach in which she wears the most fabulous sunglasses, swimsuit and turban combo – the same beach you can go to as a non-resident after paying an entrance fee! Grace also has a beautiful suite in which the couple flirt as fireworks explode outside the windows.

It's now the place to stay during the annual Film Festival and Brad Pitt, Angelina Jolie and Sharon Stone have been spotted here. In 2008 it was rumoured that Madonna refused to settle her hotel bill because a film crew had managed to get into her plush suite and film it for French TV, including the filtered water and gym equipment.

Now the bad news, it's very expensive; the Sean Connery Suite costs £12,000 a night. But off-peak some rooms can be surprisingly cheap – check out their website for deals. The Carlton Brasserie complete with gorgeous terrace is open to non-residents.

58 Boulevard la Croisette,
Cannes, France
intercontinental.com

5 CLARIDGE'S, LONDON

Movie star Spencer Tracey said, 'When I die I don't want to go to heaven, I want to go to Claridge's' and many stars feel the same way today as this hotel is their first port of call in London. It's right in the heart of Mayfair, two minutes from all the chi-chi shops in Bond Street and has a fab Champagne Bar with its own entrance on Davies Street. Here you can luxuriate in its Art Deco interior over a bottle of house bubbly – as long as you're dressed up and looking adorable. If you see photographers outside the front door (which is a common occurrence), stick around – Eva Longoria was here recently, as were Sophie Dahl, Elizabeth Hurley and Victoria Beckham. Claridge's was also the scene of Kate Moss's notorious 30th birthday party in 2004, which went on until 7.30 in the morning fuelled by strippers and Cristal champagne. Guests to *The Beautiful and The Damned* themed party included Naomi Campbell, Grace Jones, Gwyneth Paltrow and Chrissie Hynde. Kate wore a floor-length gown of blue sequins

A tip – find out what album covers the autograph hunters outside are carrying then you'll know whether it's worth waiting around. One person you won't see is Courtney Love, who was allegedly banned after accidentally starting a fire with a cigarette in 2007 – the hotel room had to be redecorated and a fireman left on duty outside her door for the rest of her stay.
Claridge's, Brook Street, London, UK
claridges.co.uk

6 CASA KIMBERLEY, PUERTO VALLARTA

Ok, so this is a little out of the way – but you need to know about it! The Casa Kimberley is a nine-bedroom bed and breakfast created out of the former homes of Richard Burton and Elizabeth Taylor. In 1964 to mark Liz's 32nd birthday Richard bought a four storeyed, ten-bedroom villa in Gringo Gulch, Puerto Vallarta for $57,000. In 1970 the couple then built another on the other side of the road for Liz to deposit

Dick in when he was one over the eight or wanted a bit of 'me time'. Dick's house had no way in or out save a pink Love Bridge that spanned the road connecting the two properties, a replica of Venice's Bridge of Sighs – also dubbed the Bridge of Reconciliations as rumour has it that after one of their wild fights they used to meet in the middle to kiss and make up. After Richard's death, Elizabeth sold the house in 1990 and was so grief stricken that she left all her personal belongings there – and they've been left exactly as they were, even down to a half finished crossword puzzle. Entering this time warp you find magazines from 1964, photographs of the couple – even a selection of Liz's clothes hanging on the wall – kaftan-tastic! You can sit in the bar personally designed by Richard and browse through their scrapbooks or visit the Cleopatra penthouse decorated in Liz's favourite shade of lavender while marvelling at her pink heart shaped bathtub. If you don't want to stay (why not, it's pretty cheap!), go on one of the tours given by the owner, who has a wealth of stories about the couple.
Casa Kimberley, Calle Zaragoza 445, Puerto Vallarta, Mexico,
casakimberley.com

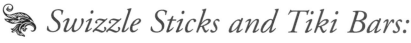

Swizzle Sticks and Tiki Bars:
A GUIDE TO GLAMOURPUSS COCKTAILS

Britney Spears may be happy to be snapped with yet another can of Red Bull grasped in her grubby paws and Sienna Miller, Gwen Stefani and Rihanna have been spotted slurping Multi V Berri Juice straight out of the bottle, but other stars are a little more elegant. Joan Crawford used to have her flasks of vodka covered in material to match her outfit. Liv Tyler likes a Strawberry Daiquiri, Kylie Minogue is partial to a Lychee Martini and Marilyn Monroe drank Dom Perignon champagne – the '53 vintage, of course! Due to their adorability many of the most famous glamourpusses had drinks named after them and they've become cocktail classics. So get the girls together, get the swizzle sticks out, put on some Xavier Cugat and have an evening of drinks Hollywood style.

'YOU SHOULD GET
out OF THOSE *wet* CLOTHES
AND INTO A *dry* MARTINI.'

Mae West

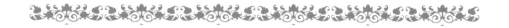

THE **MARILYN MONROE**

Take:
A quarter bottle of champagne
1½ measures apple brandy
1 teaspoon grenadine

Mix in a cocktail shaker and serve over crushed ice in a champagne saucer (the wide lipped champagne glass not the flute) with two cherries on sticks.

ELIZABETH TAYLOR'S APPLE MARTINI

Take:
1 measure vodka
1 measure apple schnapps
2 tablespoons apple juice

Pour into an ice-filled cocktail shaker, shake and then serve in a martini glass.

THE **JAYNE MANSFIELD**

Take:
2 measures vodka
3 tablespoons pineapple juice
1 tablespoon cream
1 tablespoon coconut cream
1 splash of grenadine
1 maraschino cherry, to serve

Mix all the ingredients in a cocktail shaker with crushed ice. Serve in a tall glass and top with a maraschino cherry.

THE **SOPHIA LOREN**

Take:
2 measures gin
1 tablespoon Campari
1 teaspoon Cointreau
1 teaspoon vermouth
2 tablespoons freshly squeezed
   orange juice

Coat a tall glass with the vermouth by swirling it around then pouring it out. Mix the rest of the ingredients in a cocktail shaker and then serve over crushed ice.

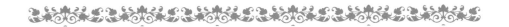

THE **MAE WEST**

Take:
1 egg yolk
1 teaspoon caster sugar
3 measures brandy
cayenne pepper, to serve

Mix together thoroughly (a little longer than normal because of the egg yolk!) and serve in a highball glass with a dash of cayenne pepper.

THE **MARLENE DIETRICH**

Take:
3 measures rye whisky
2 dashes of angostura bitters
2 dashes of curaçao
lemon peel, to serve

Mix the ingredients in a cocktail shaker and serve in a martini glass with a curl of peel on top.

THE **JEAN HARLOW**

2 measures rum
2 measures sweet Italian vermouth
lemon peel, to serve

Shake and then pour into a cocktail glass and garnish with a curl of lemon peel.

THE **GRETA GARBO** (SOMETIMES REFERRED TO AS THE GRETA GARGLE)

1 measure brandy
1 measure dry French vermouth
2 tablespoons orange juice
½ tablespoon grenadine
1 dash of crème de menthe

Shake the ingredients well and strain into a highball glass.

THE **SHIRLEY TEMPLE** (NON-ALCOHOLIC)

The world's greatest star had a drink named after her with no liquor involved (natch). It's simply a glass of ginger ale with a dash of grenadine.

✺ RIGHT: Adorability comes in all shapes and sizes and none more voluptuous than Mae West. Channel her verve by sipping on the brandy based cocktail named after her.

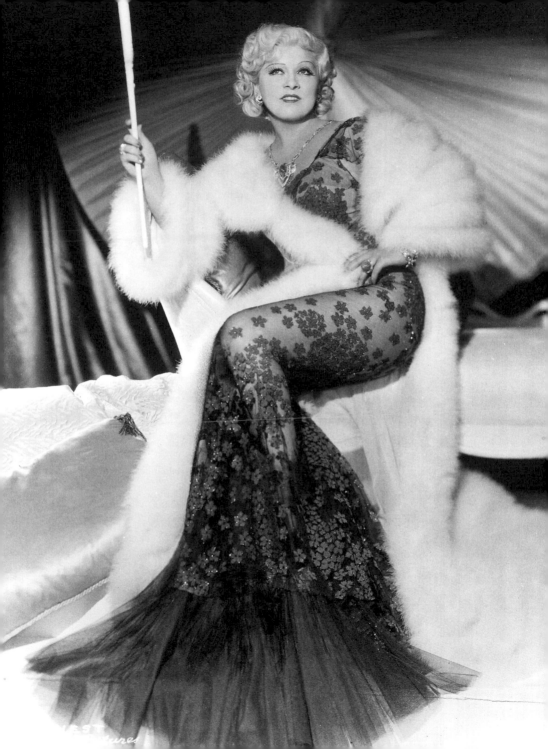

Glamour Pets: WHO HAS WHAT

To be truly adorable while posing in a hotel lobby or popping out for a quick snifter you have to have a pet. Katharine Hepburn used to walk the streets of New York with a baboon hanging from her neck and Jayne Mansfield wiggled down Sunset Boulevard with a Great Dane and an ocelot on matching leashes, both wearing huge pink bows.

Joan Crawford had a dog called Woggles and a poodle called Cliquot, who had a deluxe diet of chicken breast, ground sirloin steak and ice cream washed down with ginger ale. Joan ordered little outfits for him, too; bespoke jackets from Hammacher Schlemmer with red and black velvet collars and the dog's monogram CC (Cliquot Crawford) embroidered on them. The jackets even had tiny heart-shaped pockets with Kleenex inside in case doggie ever had to blow his nose. Most importantly Cliquot could even go from day to night with the simple application of a rhinestone collar.

Elizabeth Taylor has had a life filled with furry creatures of one kind or another, including a Maltese terrier called Sugar and a chipmunk named Nibbles when she was 14 – she even wrote a book about him, *Nibbles and Me*, that was published in 1946.

THE DACHSHUND
The chosen dog of Hollywood royalty owned by Rita Hayworth, Doris Day and Brigitte Bardot. Carole Lombard and Clark Gable had a dachshund, Commissioner, that used to blank Clark completely. After her death in 1942, however, the dog would not leave his side.

Marion Davies was so worried about her dachshund Gandhi falling into the swimming pool she had a dog friendly ladder and slide built.

➤ Perfect for drawing attention to oneself, as the dog's proportions are completely crazy.

➤ Check out how Suzanne Pleshette accessorizes with this particular brand of doggie in the 1966 movie *The Ugly Dachshund*.

THE MALTIPOO

A popular choice down Rodeo Drive as they are small and can be carried around as an accessory, rather than a sentient being. This dog is a cross between a Maltese terrier (Liz Taylor's favourite) and a poodle.

➤ Perfect for when you're wearing dark colours as it doesn't shed.

➤ Jessica Simpson owns one named Daisy.

THE HANDBAG DOG

Paris Hilton has almost single-handedly promoted this trend today with her reputed 19 miniature pooches, including the much-photographed Tinkerbell, complete with Louis Vuitton accessories. If you are prepared to go down this neon pink Swarovski-studded path (shame on you!) you will need:

➤ A copy of *The Tinkerbell Hilton Diaries: My Life Tailing Paris Hilton* (amazon.com).

➤ A hotline to Paris's range of bling for dogs, which includes a sterling silver bone-shaped pendant studded with crystals (thedivadog.com).

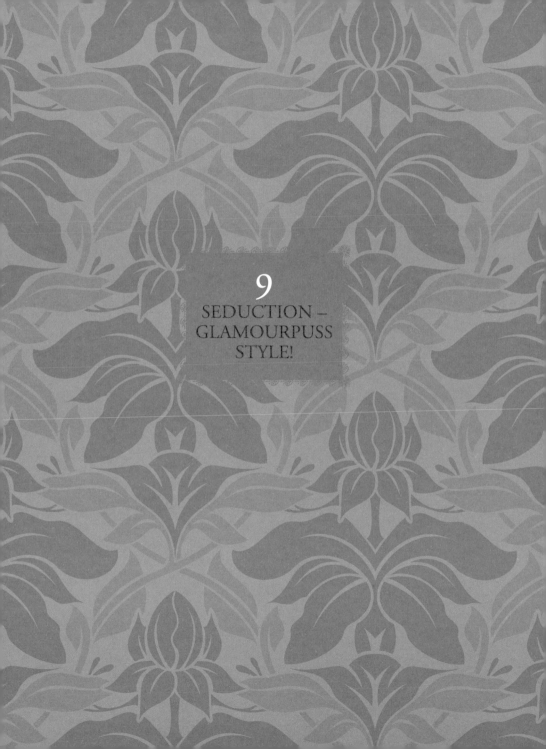

9

SEDUCTION –
GLAMOURPUSS
STYLE!

SEDUCTION – GLAMOURPUSS STYLE!

So you've dressed for success and put on your war paint, got out there and posed like a demon. Now it's time to flirt! You'll be going against contemporary mores, for it seems we are living in an era of instant sex. Nobody seems to have the time any more to start from scratch and this hit-or-miss approach to modern romance usually results in a multitude of frustrated misses and few very happy Mrs – although of course, marriage is not every woman's ultimate goal. What's all the hurry? Too much too soon can often mean a one-way ticket to unhappiness! The time is ripe to revive the lost art of flirtation.

'THE *prettiest* DRESSES ARE WORN TO BE *taken off*.'

Jean Cocteau

✳ RIGHT: Consummate flirt Kylie Minogue strikes a pose for the cameras that manages to combine seduction with style.

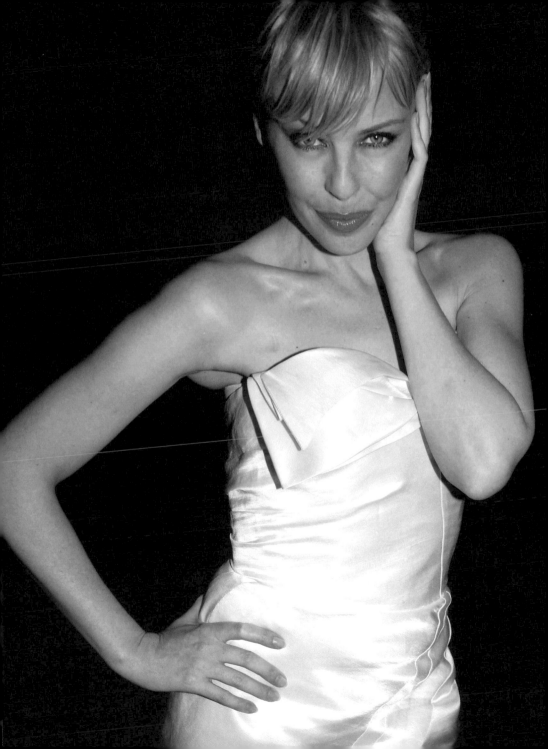

THE STREET FLIRT

If you are wiggling along the sidewalk and see a potential date striding along, make eye contact immediately. Smile, walk past but look back over your shoulder. You may well find him looking back too. If you still like the cut of his jib … STOP! Keep looking with a saucy smile. If he starts walking back, take a small step towards him and when face-to-face, arch an eyebrow and say, 'Haven't we met before?'

THE BAR FLIRT

1 Go with a group of friends including at least one man – it's easier for men to approach if there's a guy they feel they can banter with.

2 Take a trip to the ladies so you can scan the room and give all the eligible men the opportunity to feast their eyes upon you.

3 Sit at the bar so that three-quarters of your body is turned out to the room – this is your most flattering angle.

4 Talk animatedly and laugh like a tinkling bell while giving faux shy glances to your chosen one.

5 Repeat the look for a little longer, then pause, stare and smile.

6 Resume the conversation with your friends.

7 Get up and walk to the ladies again, making sure to pass by him as close as possible.

8 As you near him, raise an eyebrow. If he's interested, he'll engage you in conversation. If not, check out his mates!

DIANE BRILL'S BLANKET FLIRT THEORY
(A.K.A. THE PARTY FLIRT)

'The opportunity for flirting is everywhere so be democratic about it. Assume that every man has something you desire and employ an initial blanket flirt. Smiling to yourself as if you've just thought some whipped-cream-covered, secret sex thought is mandatory.

'Scanning a room quickly yet thoroughly and categorizing the men assembled is an essential skill that will become automatic when you practise, practise, practise! Here's the formula. Flirt – politely, with a warm smile, and welcoming glance – with 100 per cent of the men in a given room. Between 40 and 60 per cent will flirt back to some degree.

'Condense your flirt field of vision to those who flirt back. Smile and glance at members of this group, but let your attention linger on each one a second longer. About 75 per cent of these men will continue to flirt (the rest will be waiting for their dates and won't go any further).

'Narrow the group down to your lucky finalists. Find "the eyes" and lock in. Figure that a few will look away. The guys that remain are your best flirting options for the night. Pick one and flirt with him directly, but discreetly, so as not to discourage the others. Flirt with him intensely but do not monopolize his time. Excuse yourself to check out all the other finalists (or repeat the blanket-flirt process). Finally, crown the winner.'

Why I Don't Wear a Girdle
by Marilyn Monroe

'One of my own very special beauty secrets that's caused a lot of conversation [is] I don't wear a girdle – and though I say that's one of my 'secrets', it certainly is no secret from the public.

'I think the more completely natural your beauty appears to a man, the more he responds to it. And certainly that's what you're being beautiful for. I am five feet, five and a half inches in height. My hips and bust are the same – about thirty-seven. My waist is twenty-three and a half. That isn't thin – and I don't want to be. It doesn't make me look like a fashion model and I don't want to look like a fashion model.

'I personally don't happen to like the slim look a girdle gives a girl – even though I admit it does make clothes look better. And I know, almost everybody would argue with me, and tell me I'm wrong. But this just happens to be one of the things I'm stubborn about. And while I don't say it's right for everybody, I feel that it's absolutely right for me.'

Seven Sexy Movie Flirts

1959 NORTH BY NORTHWEST (dir: Alfred Hitchcock) Cary Grant and Eva Marie-Saint fall in love on a train. Her use of cigarette and matches is quite literally gripping.

1963 TOM JONES (dir: Tony Richardson) – a bit more lusty this one! There's a four-minute food orgy with no dialogue; the oyster symbolism is very naughty.

1968 THE THOMAS CROWN AFFAIR (dir: Norman Jewison) Featuring the chess scene, half lit and superbly edited – and Faye Dunaway and Steve McQueen stay vertical the whole way through.

1985 A ROOM WITH A VIEW (dir: James Ivory) Edwardian repression meets sexual tension in the romance between Helena Bonham-Carter and Julian Sands.

1986 NINE AND A HALF WEEKS (dir: Adrian Lyne) Get some lingerie tips from Kim Basinger's elegant and classy striptease for Mickey Rourke – shame about the rest of the movie, however!

1998 OUT OF SIGHT (dir: Steven Soderbergh) Jennifer Lopez and George Clooney sizzle in the boot of a car as career bank robber and female cop, recalling the sexy exchanges of Bogie and Bacall at their finest.

2001 BRIDGET JONES'S DIARY (dir: Sharon Maguire) The email flirting between Hugh Grant and Renée Zellweger is surprisingly sexy, as is his reaction to her big Spanx pants.

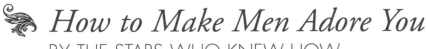

How to Make Men Adore You
BY THE STARS WHO KNEW HOW

➤ Gisele Bündchen is a famous flirt who has mastered the art of the classic hair flick. She tosses her hair to one side and exposes her gorgeous neck – a classic technique of seduction.

➤ Clara Bow said, 'Never go in for the long embrace. Pat a guy on the cheek, chuck him under his chin, fix his tie, brush an invisible speck off his lapel, or ferry a kiss from his lips to yours on your fingertips.'

➤ Tallulah Bankhead used to cartwheel knickerless in front of a prospective beau – 'I was a natural blonde and wanted to prove it.' In her later years she would whisper seductively in a lover's ear,

'KEEP LOOKING INTO MY EYES, *dahling* – MY ARSE IS LIKE AN ACCORDION – *pleated*.'

➤ Sharon Stone is perhaps a little ferocious with her prey, saying, 'Since becoming famous I get to torture a better class of man.'

➤ Lauren Bacall's mode of flirtation was dubbed 'The Look', which was created purely by accident during the screen tests for *To Have and Have Not* (1944). Bacall said, 'I used to tremble from nerves so badly that the only way I could hold my head steady was to lower my chin practically to my chest and look up at Bogie. That was the beginning of "The Look".'

✹ RIGHT: A 1945 publicity photo of Lauren Bacall sees her giving 'The Look', a seductive gaze that became her movie trademark and bagged her a Bogart.

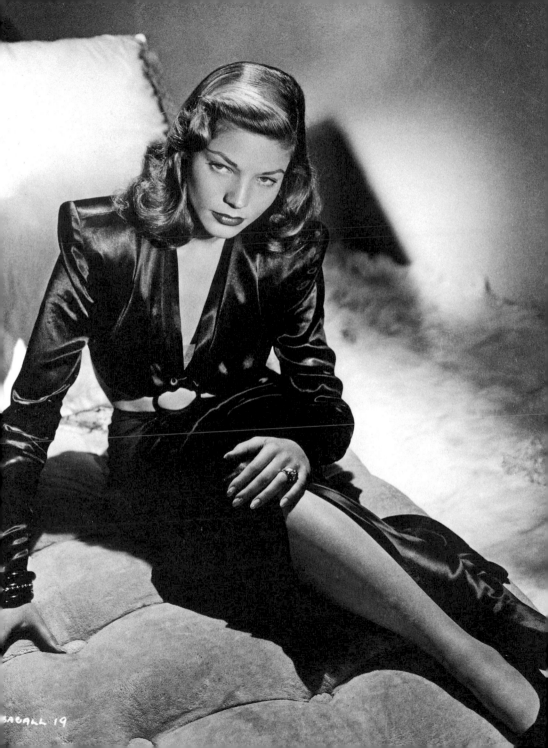

➤ Jayne Mansfield couldn't wink one eye so used to close and open both eyes whilst pouting provocatively.

➤ Kylie Minogue has a rather girlish approach:

> '*I'M* JUST A *natural flirt*, BUT I DON'T SEE IT IN A SEXUAL WAY. A LOT OF THE TIME I'M LIKE AN *over-excited puppy*.'

➤ In 2008 *Esquire* magazine named Halle Berry the sexiest woman alive. Her response? 'I don't know exactly what it means, but being 42 and having just had a baby, I think I'll take it. Sexiness is a state of mind – a comfortable state of being. It's about loving yourself in your most unlovable moments.'

➤ Drew Barrymore reads body language to find out if she's getting the green light, 'Don't listen to what he's saying. Look at what he's doing. That's so much more telling than any verbal gymnastics they're going to give you.'

➤ Socialite and diplomat Pamela Harriman was a mesmerizing seductress. She was said to have the ability to make every man she talked to think he was the centre of the universe by sitting in a pose of rapt attention. After tempting away an errant husband, his wife exclaimed, 'It was as if he had fallen into a tub of butter.'

Compare Men's Pet Hates!

Any sexual charge between man and woman will be severely muted if a little bit of you is difficult to take. In two surveys, one taken in 1965 and one in 2009 a variety of men described their biggest turn-offs when meeting women for the first time. Despite being more than 40 years apart the pet hates of the past are surprisingly similar to those of today. Budding seductresses, ignore them at your peril or you won't get past first base!

1965	2009
Obvious make-up	Too much make-up
Slip straps that show	Visible G-strings
Lipstick on cigarettes	Lipstick on teeth
Powder smears on necklines	Fake tan on sheets
Chipped nail polish	Muffin tops
Over-run heels	Cracked heels in strappy sandals
Tortured hairdos	Extensions that shed
Clanking bracelets	Piercings
Constantly looking in compact mirror	Mascara blobs in eye corners
Brassy laughter	Talking too loudly on public transport
A lumbering masculine walk	Extreme pubic waxes
Profanity	Lack of vocabulary (know what I meeean?)

❧ The Sweet Smell of Success

On your date the man will undoubtedly want to get up close and personal so you need to have the sweet smell of success about you. Remember that beauty is not just visual; it employs all of the senses. The girl who steals the spotlight in any crowd is the one who has that extra special something – a perfume that attracts men as surely as flowers attract bees. Dolores del Rio smothered herself in geranium scent, which announced her presence before she had even entered a soirée, the scent causing every man's head to swivel in her direction.

Perfume, when used with more discretion than Dolores, can be a powerful invisible ally so apply it to your pulse spots – the temple, behind the ear, at the throat, cleavage and wrists, at the bend of the arm and behind the knees.

PERFUMED STARS

When a reporter asked Marilyn Monroe, 'What do you wear in bed?' she replied, 'Chanel No. 5', a bit of cheeky repartee that rang across the world – she was also partial to Arpège by Lanvin. What did Marilyn Monroe look for in a perfume? 'Subtlety, that's what. Men like sweet scents, I believe, but they don't like to be overwhelmed by a perfume that instead of thinking of you, they are thinking, "What's that she's wearing?" Personally, I like to seek out a fragrance that isn't too popular but which is flower-like. It doesn't exude from your skin until a man is very close to you. Then when it steals over him, it is still so subtle and unfamiliar that he thinks of you, maybe not being aware of the fragrance for what it is.'

➤ CYD CHARISSE always sprayed her shoulders and hair with perfume.

➤ The 1950s French movie star CORINNE CALVET had 54 bottles to match her every mood. Her tip?

'MY *favourite* "PERFUME TRICK" IS WITH PERFUMED BATH OIL. RUB IT ALL OVER AFTER A BATH. IN 15 MINUTES THE ODOUR DISAPPEARS AS THE OIL IS ABSORBED INTO YOUR PORES. BUT LATER, WHEN YOU GO OUT, WHEN YOU ARE *dancing*, WHEN YOU GET *warm*, THE OIL IS ACTIVATED AGAIN AND THE PERFUME COMES OUT AND IS DETECTABLE AGAIN. AND THAT'S A *good time* FOR IT.'

➤ VERA MILES rinsed her lingerie in cologne-scented water.

➤ ANN SOUTHERN sprayed perfume on her petticoats so the fragrance floated about her as she walked.

➤ EVA GABOR sprayed cologne inside her lampshades so the heat of the lit bulbs diffused the fragrance subtly throughout the room.

Celebrities Talk Scents

There are many, many celebrity perfumes out there, although you can't be sure that the stars who endorse them actually wear them. The most successful is Elizabeth Taylor's White Diamonds, which since its launch in 1991 has sold more than $1billion worth. Cher's Uninhibited fared a little less well after its launch in the late 1980s and was discontinued after only a couple of years on the market – and does anyone remember Priscilla Presley's Indian Summer?

Why not do a bit of research and find out what your favourite star wears in reality. For instance, Natalie Wood, Barbara Stanwyck and Joan Crawford wore Jungle Gardenia, introduced by Tuvache in 1932. It's discontinued today but still has a huge following and vintage bottles are much sought after on ebay. Experts say that the closest to it today is Fracas by Piguet (basenotes.net). Jean Harlow and Ingrid Bergmann loved the spicy perfume Mitsouko launched by Guerlain in 1919 and still available (guerlain.com), while Katharine Hepburn wore Yves Saint Laurent's Rive Gauche (ysl-parfums.com).

Today's stars have eclectic tastes. Angelina Jolie loves Bulgari Black and has a penchant for men's cologne, Kim Cattrall wears Parure by Guerlain and Cate Blanchett Brit by Burberry. Jennifer Aniston favours the complex floral bouquet of Anaïs Anaïs that has lily as its main component, whereas Kate Winslet plumps for J'Adore, a sophisticated fragrance by Dior that has notes of mandarin, rose and violet. Salma Hayek wears Jean Paul Gaultier Classique and Elle Macpherson has used Guerlain's Vetiver for 25 years – 'I fell in love with a man who wore it and I've loved it ever since.'

Getting Ready for Your Date
by Jean Kent

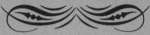

If you are tired out and have a date, don't
have a heavy meal. If you are hungry, have
a light meal before lying down. An egg
flip and cress sandwiches and a glass of
milk or tomato soup would be nourishing
and easy to digest. Perhaps some kind
person would bring a tray up to your
bedroom; most mothers are perfect jewels
in this respect. Now, having undressed and
drawn the curtains, lie on the bed, put two
pads of cotton wool soaked in Optrex on
each eye and relax. If you can sleep, so
much the better. After 30 minutes you will
feel quite refreshed and looking forward to
your date. A few favourite bath salts in
your bath, a good towelling, and heigh
ho, you are ready for the high spots.

The Boudoir

You have flirted successfully and captured your prey. If you feel the time is right, dim the lights and set the scene for seduction. Prepare for a night of passion!

Your boudoir has to create a *mise en scène* of erotic enchantment, a shop window in which you are the most alluring ware – think chandelier, a pink satin throw and matching headboard. Sparkling Venetian mirrors should be dotted around to reflect your libidinous poses and a touch of zebra skin (faux, of course) helps to set the mood.

Modern women don't have to be fey and submissive but we can still take advice. Elise de Wolf suggested that an aquarium full of fan-tailed goldfish next to the bed and a small gold lacquer Chinese pagoda containing a pet chihuahua would create the right exotic ambience for the sexy femme fatale. Jean Harlow lay on a shell-shaped bed in white satin, and Jayne Mansfield reclined in pastel pleasure in her Pink Palace on Sunset Boulevard. Her fantasy 1950s boudoir was all leopard-skin throws and powder puffs, a place to drink from a pink champagne fountain illuminated by gold cupids festooned with fluorescent lights.

Your boudoir should be a stage set too, bedecked with crystal chandeliers and tiger skin rugs where you reign supreme mixing dry Martinis for each besotted suitor. Props should include Merry Widow corsets, seamed stockings and suspenders. For an authentic vintage feel source a blond wood dressing table and matching quilted boudoir chair on which you can sit, unfurl your chiffon robe and peel down your seamed stockings with the right degree of seductive suggestion.

And pink, that most obviously feminine of colours, should run riot – rose pink, blush, shocking and fuschia – a colour frivolous and fluffy, a perfect complement to taffeta, net and lace.

THE MARABOU MULE

A boudoir *mise en scène* is incomplete without a pair of fluffy marabou mules – especially erotic when you cross your legs and allow one to dangle suggestively off your naked foot. The best were made in the 1950s by Frederick's of Hollywood – their Bareback Mule as worn by pin-up Bettie Page and Cyd Charisse was legendary. It came in zebra print, red or black patent or lucite studded with pink rhinestones. *Ooh là là!*

Frederick's mules remain the best on the market today, in particular the Glamour Girl Marabou Slipper (only $30ish), which comes complete with a satin vamp and three inch heel – they also do a sexy Glamour Girl Lace Slipper for the same price in red, black and white. Frederick's Fantasy outfits are also worth a peek (for a little later in your relationship). They're a hoot in a modern burlesque kind of way and the Sultry Sailor and Shanghai Girl have a real retro feel about them. Check out the Bunny Girl, Fräulein (complete with beer stein) and Exotic Belly Dancer, too. (fredericks.com)

HOW TO
Undress *for a Man*

The lingerie a woman chooses sends a powerful message about who she is and the potency of her sexual power. It's easy to enjoy the sensuality of your own body if you cover it in the most delicate of materials; soft satins and chiffon that touch it like your lover's caress. As supermodel Elle Macpherson, a.k.a. The Body, put it,

> 'IF YOU'RE WEARING *lingerie* THAT MAKES YOU *feel* GLAMOROUS, YOU'RE HALFWAY THERE TO *turning heads*.'

You must never deny yourself lovely lingerie even if only the very special few will see it – it will make you feel differently about yourself. It's important to realize that you don't need the body of a model to wear lingerie, it can be used to enhance the parts you're proud of and disguise the bits that are slightly alarming. And if you're wearing a gorgeous pair of antique rose French knickers trimmed with Valençiennes lace or a black chiffon peignoir, there's no way anyone, male or female, will be looking at your cellulite! Let's face it, we all have it, 'even supermodels' says actress Sandra Bullock: 'I've been to fashion shows and seen it. It's nature. Without it you aren't human.' And take a tip from Sarah Jessica Parker; she uses body lotion on the front part of her shins to get eye-catching shimmering legs – another trick to draw the eye away from so-called problem areas.

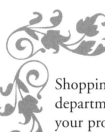

Shopping for lingerie is easy these days as most department stores have fitters who can tell you your proper bra size – and there are many online boutiques that sell a range of international designer brands. Among the best are:

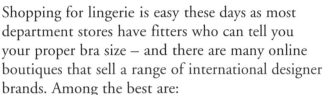

agentprovocateur.com – a high end fashion forward brand, founded by Joe Corre and Serena Rees in 1994, which combines retro glamour with catwalk chic.

bravissimo.com – stocks larger sizes for curvier bodies. It has excellent fitting information.

damaris.co.uk – a beautiful label that specializes in display rather than practicality. Angelina Jolie and Kirsten Dunst have shopped here, and this is the site to buy gorgeous fripperies such as waspies fashioned out of wisps of black lace and Damaris's signature bow-back panties designed to give maximum cleavage to your delicious derrière.

figleaves.com – a popular website for good reason, it has a huge range of brands.

glamonweb.com – the home of deluxe brand La Perla.

glamorousamorous.com – lots of leopard-print and marabou trim – Grrrrr!

lingerieatlarge.com – large sizes and saucy styles!

❧ *Stars* Uncovered

HALLE BERRY inadvertently let slip about her underwear in an interview about the prospects of her latest film. 'What's the worst that can happen? If it doesn't do well, I can put on my big-girl panties, deal with it and move on.'

LUPE VELEZ didn't need such unnatural enhancements – her huge breasts, described by Errol Flynn as 'the most beautiful in Hollywood', were regularly displayed at Tinseltown bashes when she used to rotate them one at a time!

MARILYN MONROE eliminated underwear because she felt that panty lines distracted from her shapely rear – as she put it, 'All those lines and ridges in undergarments are unnatural and they distort a girl, so I never wear them.'

JANE RUSSELL had a bra engineered for her by Howard Hughes for her appearance in the movie *The Outlaw* in 1943. Hughes gave Russell such an audacious cleavage that the movie was banned until 1950. At the long-awaited premiere, when Jane leaned over provocatively, a member of the audience shouted 'Bombs Away!'

JAYNE MANSFIELD abandoned bras when she was 14 in order 'to be free'. As she put it coquettishly, 'I hate under-things!' Often one breast would suddenly pop out of her strapless gowns for the benefit of the Hollywood paparazzi.

✻ RIGHT: Halle Berry uses her orange bikini worn in the James Bond movie *Die Another Day* to see if she's put on any weight by trying it on every couple of months to make sure it still fits. 'If I can't get into it, I eat less junk food for a bit. It's really useful.'

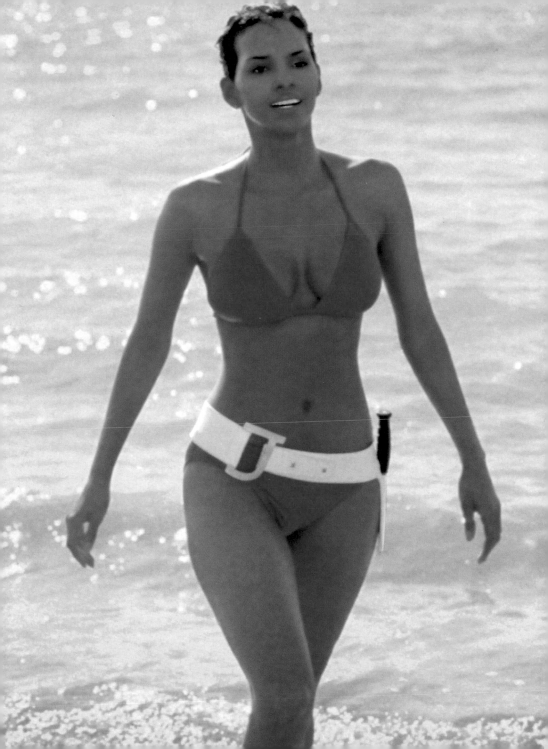

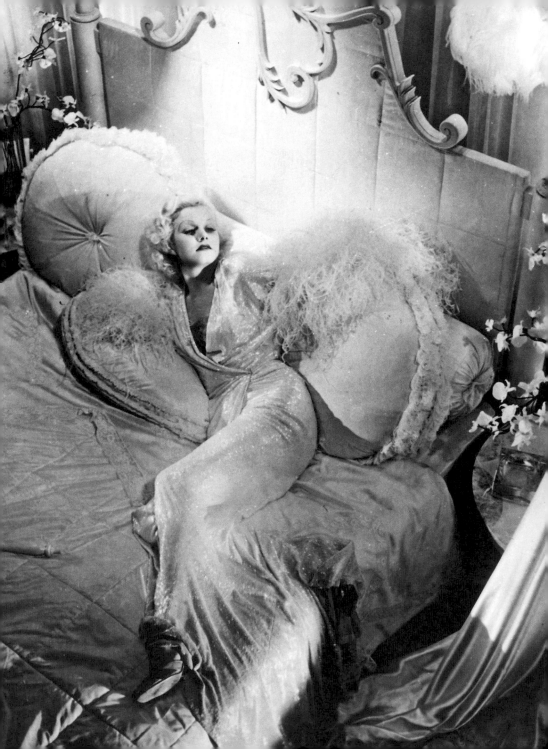

Like Cameron Diaz, JEAN HARLOW was famed for her no bra look which she emphasized by wearing bias-cut satin gowns by famed Hollywood designer Adrian, cut to cling to the curves of her voluptuous body. Jean's white satin gowns were so tight she wore no underwear and had to bleach her pubic hair so that it didn't show through. Nothing seemed to lie beneath her dresses and her skin save a little filmy perspiration. Jean's repartee at press conferences was flirtatious in the extreme:

'Jean, would you advise a young woman to take a lover instead of a husband?'
I'd advise her to take what she can get – and to keep on shopping.'
'Why do you think audiences like you, Miss Harlow?'
'The men like me because I don't wear a brassière. And women like me because I don't look like the kind of girl who would steal a husband. At least not for long.'
'But would you steal a husband, Miss Harlow?'
'Wouldn't that be like shopping in a secondhand store?'
'Are you wearing a brassière now, Miss Harlow?'
'That sounds like a near-sighted question.'

After arriving in Hollywood, breathy blonde glamourpuss JUDY HOLLIDAY was taken to the studio's make-up and costume departments to be tweaked. Afterwards, she vamped into the boss's office and he was so overcome with lust that he lunged – whereupon one of her falsies popped out of her dress and bounced onto the floor, 'That's all right,' she quipped, 'It's yours anyway.'

My Stocking Technique
by Kathleen Hughes

Nylons are precious, delicate things that deserve the best of care, whether you have one pair or a dozen. In Hollywood we look after our stockings with particular care. We have a special technique in the way we put on our stockings so as to keep them free from ladders and snags.

1 Always roll a stocking down right to the tip of the toe before inserting the foot. This prevents toenails from snagging the material.

2 When drawing on the stocking, slowly unroll it over the foot, keeping the thumbs on the back seam to keep the stocking straight.

3 Keeping thumbs close against the seam, gently draw the stocking up the leg, keeping the seam straight so there's no need to pull it up and stretch it later.

4 Anchor your stockings securely to your suspender belt or girdle.

5 Take one last look to check the seams in the mirror.

Love *in the Afternoon*
– CINQ À SEPT

The French have always had a reputation as seasoned seducers and Paris as a glittering city of erotic pleasure, never more so than during La Belle Epoque, the name given to the last decade of the nineteenth century – a decade that now has a reputation as sparkling as vintage champagne. Women were erotic queens whose clothes whispered with innuendo and presented their bodies as delicious packages to be unwrapped. Cascading petticoats rustled suggestively as they were drawn up the thighs by bewitched suitors, and there were many unwritten codes that had to be followed by those who expected to enjoy the pleasures of the flesh.

A custom that dates from those times and still exists today is the *cinq à sept*, the period of from five to seven pm that is set aside for married men and women to discreetly meet their lovers and then dash home for a 7.30 dinner with a more official partner. In the 1890s these assignations had to be organized with military precision as it was considered ill-bred for a woman to walk along the city streets without a chaperone. Coachmen had to be instructed to take the eager participants to an arranged meeting place and then to turn a blind eye to the sexual shenanigans within.

Once inside her bower of love, a woman had seriously to consider how to undress and dress without the aid of her usual maid as clothing was constricting, complicated and difficult to get on and off. It wouldn't take much for a husband to work out if he was being made a fool –

an inexpertly laced corset at bedtime, perhaps, or a button come adrift. One French coquette was forced to lay out a specific set of plans for her rich lover, informing him,

> '_IF YOU WANT ME TO undress, I must HAVE A MAID TO HELP ME. AND that's not all! I WARN YOU THAT I DON'T KNOW HOW TO DO MY OWN HAIR SO I must HAVE A coiffeur, PREFERABLY FROM LENTHERIC, TO ARRANGE IT._'

Aware that the date was proving to be a little more expensive than anticipated, her lover tried to cut costs by stressing that he wouldn't dream of mussing up her hairstyle. Her saucy retort 'Don't guarantee on me remaining immobile during our passionate romp!'

In the 1960s the time for illicit romance subtly shifted to between two and four pm as traffic in most French cities ground to a standstill and men and women found it too difficult to leave their lovers and get home on time. But swinging 1960s fashions had their use for the bored housewife itching to meet a swarthy gigolo. The fashion for wigs in this decade meant she could make a fictitious hair appointment and send the wig instead. After the afternoon's romp, the wig was worn to dinner with the wife appearing perfectly coiffed in front of her unsuspecting husband.

Today it's back to *cinq à sept* again, a time of the day to look forward to with a delicious frisson of anticipation during a routine office meeting. It's easier to create an alibi these days with longer working hours, and modern women can plead pressure at work for their late arrival at suppertime. Today's uncomplicated hairstyles make it simpler to pack a pair of GHDs to straighten the hair after an afternoon of eroticism. The simplest hairstyle to avoid deception is the mussed-up bedhead look usually sported by Kate Moss. Keep make-up to a minimum so that it can be re-applied with ease after your assignation – brighten underneath the eyes with peach-toned concealer and powder your T-zone. Add a little touch of mascara and a dab of clear lip gloss.

The best outfit for a *cinq à sept* has to be the wrap dress – easy to put on and pull off in one and cut to flatter the body's curves in a subtly sexy and elegant way. This classic design was created by Diane von Furstenberg in 1974 at the height of feminism and seemed to encapsulate the new freedom that women were feeling in the same way as Yves Saint Laurent was incorporating elegant simplicity and sexuality for the new women of Europe. By 1976 millions of wrap dresses had been sold. Since its relaunch in 1997 this signature style has maintained its popularity. The wrap's combination of elegance and allure exudes the adult sophistication needed for the *cinq à sept* – one mustn't look as if trying too hard and too much powder, paint, leather and lace is inappropriate for day wear – and a little too obvious! It's about whispering, not screaming, sexuality.

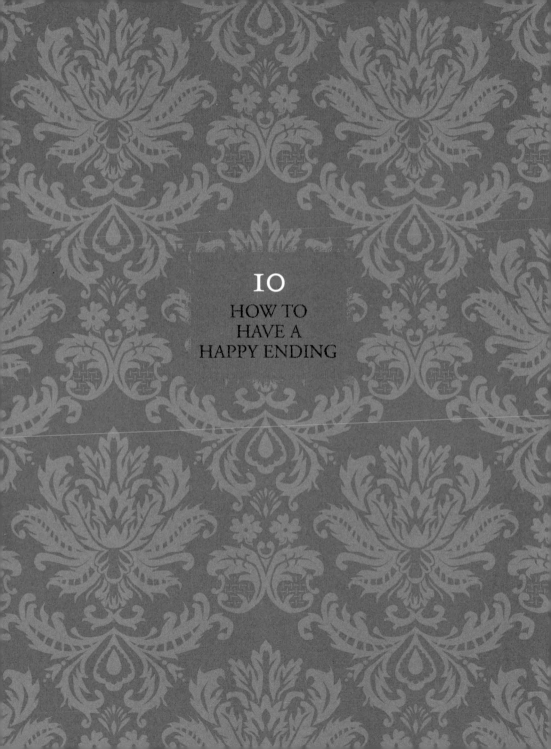

IO

HOW TO
HAVE A
HAPPY ENDING

HOW TO HAVE
A HAPPY ENDING

Your happy ending can be breakfast and goodbye or
something a little more permanent. Today we have that
choice. A happy ending can of course mean one couple
entwined for all eternity but it can also mean a good career
with no children, following in the footsteps of the sublime
Helen Mirren, or a series of rich and powerful men like
Jackie O. It could mean multiple marriages and a disgraceful
old age like Liz Taylor, or spending all your money in the
casinos of Monte Carlo with a toy boy *comme* Colette.
Juliette Binoche manages successfully to combine single
parenthood with a son and daughter born to different fathers
and an internationally acclaimed career. 'Giving birth is like
a vase of beautiful flowers,' she says. 'Only you're just the
vase, and only for a very short moment. The flowers are
beautiful, but they belong to themselves, not to the vase.'

So, the choice is yours – as Katharine Hepburn said, 'If you
want to sacrifice the admiration of many men for the
criticism of one – go ahead, get married.' The key to any
happy ending, though, is adorability. No matter what you
decide, or what the fates thrust upon you, if you love and are
loved in return your ending will a be happy one.

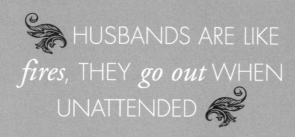

HUSBANDS ARE LIKE *fires*, THEY *go out* WHEN UNATTENDED

Zsa Zsa Gabor

🪶 *The* Morning After *Breakfast*

It's the morning after and if you feel the required duties have been performed with the right degree of enthusiasm, athleticism and aplomb it's time to show off your skills in the kitchen (or if not, just send him on his way with the bus fare and a bacon buttie).

Grace Kelly favoured yogurt and honey, Greta Garbo rye bread and cheese – whatever floats your boat. And if in doubt, eat out – in 2006 Kate Hudson and on-off lover Owen Wilson shared a breakfast of scrambled egg with tofu and banana pancakes at an organic restaurant in Los Angeles; Reese Witherspoon and Jake Gyllenhaal ate omelette and fruit and read the *Los Angeles Times* together at Le Pain Quotidien in Brentwood, California, in 2008.

Not all of us have such top-notch eateries in our immediate environs, though – Chubby's, Chicken Cottage and Kebab Planet spring to mind – so try some of these glamourpuss breakfast ideas instead:

ARLENE DAHL'S
EGGS DAHLIA
4 eggs
4 tablespoons milk or cream
1 teaspoon beef stock powder
1 teaspoon fresh grated Parmesan
  cheese
salt and pepper
1 spring onion, finely chopped
25g/1oz butter
handful of parsley, finely chopped

Combine the eggs, milk, stock powder
and cheese. Whip them up with a fork.
Add the salt, pepper and spring onion.
Melt the butter in a hot frying pan and
pour in the egg mixture. When it begins
to set slightly, lower the flame and stir
occasionally. Don't allow the mixture to
stick to the bottom. While the eggs are
still soft and loose, turn them out on to
a warm plate, and garnish with parsley.
Serve with toast and bacon or sausage.

MAE WEST'S
HEALTHY BREAKFAST
1 large banana
1 large apple
1 large pear
200ml/7fl oz milk
1 tablespoon runny honey
1 tablespoon chopped almonds

Chop up the fruit, pour in the milk and
drizzle with honey. Sprinkle with the
chopped almonds and serve.

SOPHIA LOREN'S
COURGETTE OMELETTE
4 tablespoons olive oil
115g/4oz courgettes, thinly sliced
6 eggs
salt and pepper
1 tablespoon chopped parsley

Heat half the olive oil in a large frying
pan and gently fry the courgettes until
soft. Meanwhile, whisk the eggs and
season with salt and pepper. Stir the
parsley and cooked courgettes into the
eggs. Heat the remaining olive oil in the
frying pan and add the egg and
courgette mixture. Cook until the
underside is crisp, then serve warm.

Breakfast at Marilyn's

By nature I have a languorous disposition.
I hate to do things in a hurried tense
atmosphere and it is virtually impossible for
me to spring out of bed in the morning.
On Sunday, which is my day of total leisure,
I sometimes take two hours to wake up,
luxuriating in every last drop of drowsiness.
Depending upon my activities, I sleep
between five and ten hours a night. I have
never been able to wear pajamas or creepy
nightgowns; they disturb my sleep.

'Before I take my morning shower, I start
warming a cup of milk on a hot plate. When
it's hot I break two raw eggs into the milk,
whip them up with a fork and drink them
while I'm dressing. I supplement this with a
multi-vitamin pill and I doubt if any doctor
could recommend a more nourishing
breakfast for a working girl in a hurry.

HOW TO GIVE HIM THE BRUSH-OFF

The easiest way? Just don't return his calls, then he can make up any excuse to save face such as your sudden emigration to Botswana or your inability to cope with his huge … sexual demands. If you are brave enough to do it face-to-face (unlike Matt Damon, who told Minnie Driver they had split on *The Oprah Winfrey Show*), you can tell him that you really like him – but your probation officer doesn't. Or to send him really running and screaming for the hills? 'I want you, I need you. Let's get married and have babies!'

THE GIRL THAT I MARRY BY FARLEY GRANGER

'First of all, let me get one thing straight. I am a guy who likes one girl. I don't "play the field". Once I find a girl I like to be with, then I'm satisfied to stay with her for as long as our friendship lasts. I don't "date" a different girl every night. That's not the way I work. The girl that I marry should be a pal first and foremost. I don't want to marry someone and then put them on a pedestal. I want a real down-to-earth human being, with a sense of humour, a keen sense of fun and an appreciation of life. I want to marry a girl with whom I can share everything – my likes, my dislikes, my sorrows, my joys. I want a girl with understanding, a girl who has time to listen to other people's troubles. She may be beautiful. And then again she may not be. I like a girl for the way she talks, the way she walks, the neat way she dresses and the gay colours she wears, the way her hair shines and the way her nose crinkles when she smiles. I like her to laugh a lot and to find a lot to enjoy in life. I'm a gay person myself and I'd like the girl I marry to be the same.'

Wedding Daze

Weddings are more popular than ever, even though they are increasingly likely to fail. And stars are prepared to spend spectacularly to achieve the right effect. On July 29th 1981 a nation drowned in sugar syrup as Diana Spencer entered Saint Paul's Cathedral wearing an ivory silk taffeta dress designed by David and Elizabeth Emanuel with a twenty-five foot detachable court train and loose full sleeves caught at the elbow with taffeta bows. Victoria and David Beckham's 'low-key affair', as their spokesperson put it, involved 300 guests flown in to Luttrellstown Castle, a 560-acre estate near Dublin, for a reception costing a million dollars during which they posed on lurid gold thrones.

But perhaps the most ostentatious (and bizarre) ceremony was the renewal of wedding vows by Céline Dion and René Angélil in 2000. The Ballroom of Caesar's Palace in Las Vegas was decorated in the style of *The Arabian Nights* and an estimated $1.5 million spent on Berber tents, circus performers and imported camels forming the backdrop to Dion, who was carried in reclining on a white chaise longue. At the end of the ceremony the happy bride and groom were crowned.

TIP Themed weddings *can* be cool but try to avoid nerdy ones with a *Star Wars* theme or anything from Walt Disney. Remember, those photos are going to be around for ever. One wonders if Trudie Styler and Sting cringe when flicking through their wedding photo album to see snaps of the Versace white and gold 'Victorian' gown, a monstrous concoction that managed to scream '80s!' in 1992.

Fab Five Wedding Movies

1. SEX AND THE CITY: THE MOVIE (2008 dir: Michael Patrick King) The mother of all wedding movies that stresses it's about the man, not the dress (but it gives plenty of opportunities to lust after gowns designed by Vivienne Westwood, Caroline Herrera, Lacroix, Dior and Oscar de la Renta on the way).

2. HIGH SOCIETY (1956 dir: Charles Walters) Grace Kelly marries Bing Crosby (a man whose proposal she had turned down in real life) wearing a lavender crinoline and picture hat by Helen Rose.

3. FOUR WEDDINGS AND A FUNERAL (1994 dir: Mike Newell) Commitment-phobe Charlie (Hugh Grant) and the mysterious Carrie (Andie MacDowell) form a relationship and fall in love during other people's weddings.

4. 27 DRESSES (2008 dir: Anne Fletcher) Katherine Heigl is always the bridesmaid and shows the true theme of a themed wedding – humiliation.

5. FATHER OF THE BRIDE (1950) Deliberately scheduled to open a month after Elizabeth Taylor's real-life marriage to Nicky Hilton (Uncle of celebutante Paris Hilton). The nuptial splendour of Liz's sweetheart-line gown is totally gorgeous!

➤ GRACE KELLY's wedding gown, designed by Helen Rose, was made from 98 yards of tulle, 25 yards of silk taffeta and 300 yards of lace. Her veil was covered in a web of thousands of seed pearls with a motif of lovebirds appliquéd in lace.

➤ With eight wedding ceremonies behind her, ELIZABETH TAYLOR is one of the most married and divorced glamourpusses in the world. As comedian Spike Milligan joked,

> 'I REMEMBER MY BROTHER ONCE SAYING, *"I'd like to marry Elizabeth Taylor"* AND MY FATHER SAID, *"Don't worry, son your turn will come".'*

➤ At her 1964 marriage to Richard Burton in Montreal Liz wore a yellow chiffon décolleté gown based on the one she had worn for her first scenes with Richard in *Cleopatra* – all the better to show off the diamond necklace he'd given her. Her hair was bulked out with $600 worth of Italian hairpieces that were woven through with white Roman hyacinths, all references to the place where they had first met. Best friend Oscar Levant joked, 'Always a bride never a bridesmaid.' Burton started drinking at 10am and was pretty unsteady on his feet, moving Liz to quip, 'I don't know why he's so nervous. We've been sleeping together for two years.'

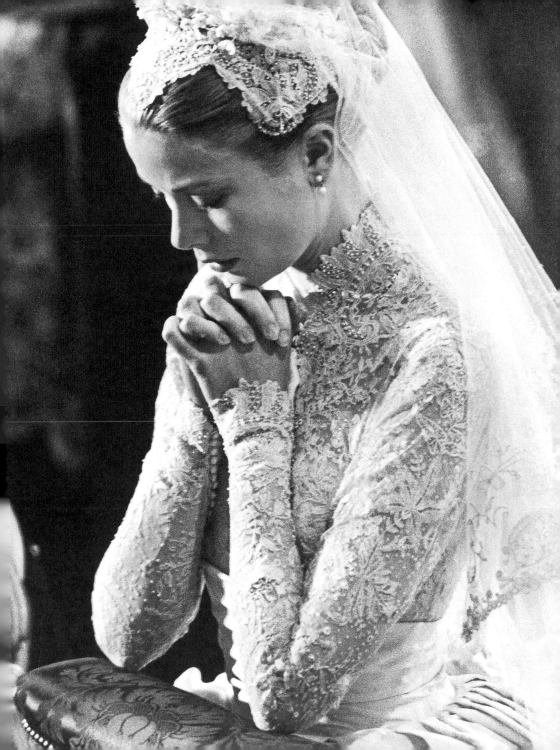

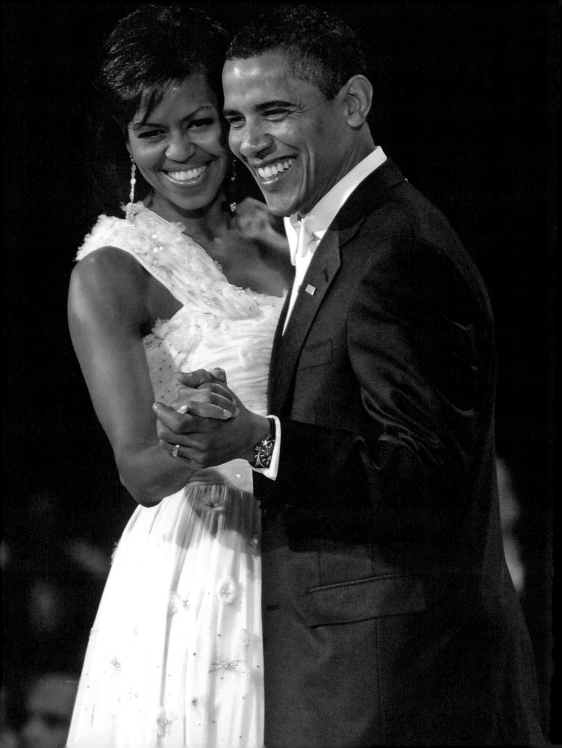

➤ After two years of dating Barack Obama, feisty MICHELLE OBAMA was getting a bit cheesed off about his intellectual theorizing on whether marriage was a relevant or anachronistic institution in modern culture. In 1991 over dinner at a swish restaurant she told him to shape up or ship out. A dessert arrived, she noticed a box and opened it up – it was an engagement ring! 'That kind of shuts you up, doesn't it?' smirked Obama. When asked in 2004 after 15 years of happy union what the dessert was, Michelle Obama replied, 'I don't even remember. I don't think I even ate it. I was so shocked, and sort of a little embarrassed, because he did sort of shut me up.'

➤ In 2000 CATHERINE ZETA-JONES wore an Edwardian-inspired gown by French couturier Christian Lacroix that cost $160,000. It was made of ivory duchesse satin with a long 1930s fishtail skirt overlaid with 18th-century Chantilly lace and a seven-foot train.

➤ As guests left SARAH JESSICA PARKER and Matthew Broderick's wedding in 1997 they were given a piece of wedding cake with a note, 'Put this under your pillow and dream of your true love.'

➤ In 1935 writer COLETTE married at the age of 63. It was her third time – the groom Maurice Gondekat was 45. The wedding party feasted on pork knuckles and pancakes at a country inn.

➤ During WALLIS SIMPSON's marriage to Edward VIII, celebrity crimper Antoine flew his plane overhead to drop thousands of white lilies from the sky.

❦ *How to Make It* Last

How about some more specific advice to keep the flames of love, and indeed desire, burning? Christina Aguilera recommends naturism, something most of us associate with middle-aged couples in caravan parks displaying their dangly bits during an energetic game of badminton! She reveals that she and her husband Jordan Bratman

'HAVE SOMETHING CALLED *naked Sundays*. YOU HAVE TO KEEP MARRIAGE ALIVE, *spice it up*. WE DON'T NEED TO GO *anywhere*. WE'RE JUST WITH EACH OTHER. WE DO *everything naked*. WE *cook naked*.'

Catherine Zeta-Jones believes that 'for marriage to be a success, every woman and every man should have their own bathroom'. And Jerry Hall? 'My mother said it was simple to keep a man. You must be a maid in the living room, a cook in the kitchen and a whore in the bedroom. I said I'd hire the other two and take care of the bedroom bit.'

Joanne Woodward and Paul Newman were married for 50 years before his death in 2008. They met at a theatrical agency in New York – he was 27 and she was 22. On their marriage Paul presented his new wife with a silver cup inscribed:

SO YOU WOUND UP WITH APOLLO
IF HE'S SOMETIMES HARD TO SWALLOW
USE THIS.

Their daughter Nell was born in 1959, Melissa in 1961, and Clea in 1964. The couple lived simply in Connecticut, far away from the temptations of glitzy Hollywood – and Newman was known for travelling everywhere with a flask of his wife's coffee. When asked how their marriage had lasted, Paul said, 'I've repeatedly said that for people who have as little in common as Joanne and myself, we have an uncommonly good marriage. Husbands and wives should have separate interests, cultivate different sets of friends and not impose on the other … You can't spend a lifetime breathing down each other's necks … We are very, very different people and yet somehow we fed off those varied differences and instead of separating us, it has made the whole bond a lot stronger.' Joanne Woodward put it more succinctly:

> '*Sexiness wears thin* AFTER A WHILE AND *beauty fades*, BUT TO BE MARRIED TO A MAN WHO MAKES YOU *laugh every day*, AH, NOW THAT'S A *real treat.*'

Simone Signoret said, 'Chains do not hold a marriage together. It is threads, hundreds of tiny threads which sew people together through the years. That is what makes a marriage last – more than passion or even sex!' Good advice because she was married to French singer and actor Yves Montand for 34 years – despite his short-lived affair with Marilyn Monroe. Her response? A dignified 'She will never know how much I never hated her.'

Liz Taylor
Muses on Marriage

'My mother says I didn't open my eyes for eight days after I was born, but when I did, the first thing I saw was an engagement ring. I was hooked.'

'Your heart knows when you've met the right man. There is no doubt that Nicky is the one I want to spend my life with.' They divorced ten months later.

'I am a very committed wife. And I should be committed, too – for marrying so many times.'

'I've only slept with men I've been married to. How many women can make that claim?'

'Richard is a very sexy man. He's got that sort of jungle essence that one can sense.'

☀ RIGHT: Elizabeth Taylor with husband no. 4, Eddie Fisher. He said of her, 'Sexually she was every man's dream; she had the face of an angel and the morals of a truck driver.'

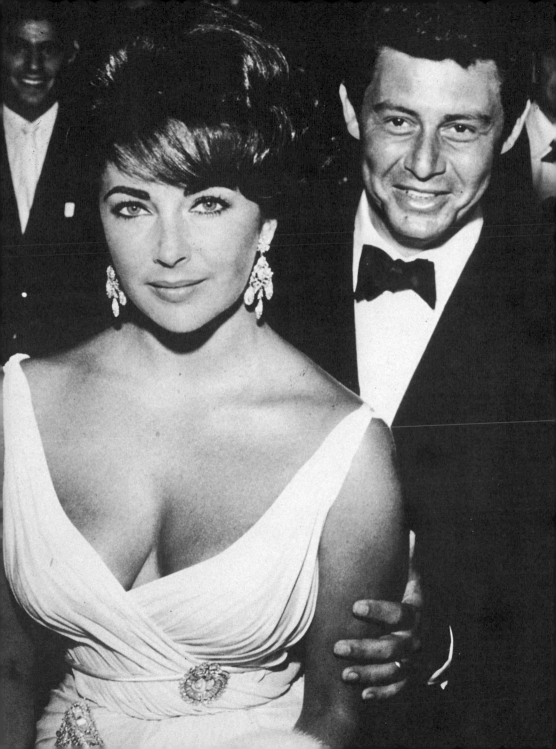

How to be Married, Single, Whatever ... and Happy!

➤ KIM CATTRALL as Samantha in *Sex and The City* survives in a sea of schmaltz. After a five year relationship with Smith Jerrod, she realizes she's happier single, saying, 'I love you – but I love me more.' Art mimics life for Cattrall, who has been married and divorced three times, written a book on the female orgasm and been linked with a string of gorgeous men.

➤ TALLULAH BANKHEAD: 'I'm not childless, dahling. I'm child-free.' Openly bisexual, Tallulah was linked with many famous names including Greta Garbo and Marlene Dietrich, and was renowned for getting drunk and stripping off at parties. She died unrepentant at the age of 66 – her last words, 'Codeine! Bourbon!'

➤ CARLA BRUNI: 'Love lasts a long time, but burning desire – two to three weeks.' Love seems to have lasted with this model turned musician turned First Lady of France. Bruni met and married French Prime Minister Nicolas Sarkozy in 2008 after a rackety love life that included Mick Jagger and Eric Clapton. Karl Lagerfeld described the couple's first meeting as like that of 'hunters ... predators. He had seduced many women and she was a seductress. When two like this meet, it can be good.'

➤ SCARLETT JOHANSSON is equally practical. 'I don't think that monogamy is a natural instinct for human beings. Monogamy can be hard work for some people. You don't always meet the right person at the right time.' In 2008 she married the actor Ryan Reynolds at the remote Clayoquot wilderness resort in Vancouver famed for its 'glamping' – that's glamorous camping to you and me.

➤ HEDY LAMARR was married six times and remained a rebel to the end at the age of 87: 'Some men like a dull life – they like the routine of eating breakfast, going to work, coming home, petting the dog, watching TV, kissing the kids, and going to bed. Stay clear of it – it's often catching.'

➤ KATHARINE HEPBURN: 'Sometimes I wonder if men and women really suit each other. Perhaps they should live next door and just visit now and then' – an apt description of her own long-running relationship with fellow actor Spencer Tracy, which ended only with his death in 1967.

➤ BEYONCÉ KNOWLES:

'THERE'S *definitely* A DANGEROUS FEELING WHEN YOU'RE *in love* – IT'S GIVING YOUR HEART TO SOMEONE ELSE AND KNOWING THAT THEY HAVE *control* OVER YOUR FEELINGS. I KNOW FOR ME, WHO *always* TRIES TO BE SO TOUGH, THAT'S THE *dangerous* THING.'

Beyoncé married longtime-love rapper Jay-Z in a refreshingly top secret ceremony in New York in 2008.

➤ ZSA ZSA GABOR: 'A man in love is incomplete before he's married. Then he's finished', and 'Getting divorced just because you don't love a man is almost as silly as getting married just because you do.' Born in 1917, Gabor has been married and divorced a breathtaking nine times.

➤ BETTE DAVIS: After surviving four failed marriages she remarked, 'I'd marry again if I found a man who had 15 million dollars and would sign over half of it to me before the marriage, and guarantee he'd be dead within the year.'

➤ CHER: 'The trouble with some women is that they get all excited about nothing – and then marry him.' She's only been married twice, fairly tame by Hollywood standards and in 2008 admitted that she was currently dating three much younger men in rotation. Her net wealth is reckoned to be $1 billion.

➤ REESE WITHERSPOON says, 'Many people worry so much about managing their careers, but rarely spend half that much energy managing their LIVES. I want to make my life, not just my job, the best it can be. The rest will work itself out.'

And when looking back over your *own* blooming, tortured or lacklustre love life, always remember the wise words of Carrie Bradshaw: 'Some love stories aren't epic novels, they're short stories – but that doesn't make them any less filled with love.'

Don't be a Slipshod Woman!
by Jean Kent

If we get slack at home, when we
are married we may slip into the old
habit, and one thing most men loathe is a
slip-shod woman. We dressed and groomed
ourselves to win our man; we must dress
and groom ourselves to keep him. If not,
we must not grumble if he casts admiring
glances at some attractive girl. Once a man
finds that a girl does not care whether she
is attractive or smart, a beautiful ideal dies.
A man once told me that if only women
realized how much their husbands hope
that their wives will never sink to 'dressing
up' only when they are going out, she would
do anything rather than let him
see her untidy or unattractive.

References

p.6 Gwyneth Paltrow in http://cosmo.intoday.in/cosmopolitan/story.jsp?sid=6676

p.11 Lilly Daché, *Lilly Daché's Glamour Book*. (Philadelphia: J. B. Lippincoff, 1956), p.6

p.12 Marilyn Monroe on Peter Noble and Yvonne Saxon, *Glamour: Film, Fashion and Beauty* (London: Burke, 1953), p.5

p.13 Ibid., p.3

p.13 Arthur Miller, 'The Power and the Glamour' in *Allure*, April, 2002

p.16 Angelina Jolie in brainyquote.com/quotes/authors/a/angelina_jolie.html

p.19 Gwen Stefani in thinkingheadsinc.com/People/Quotations/tabid/106/Default.aspx

p.19 Arlene Dahl, *Always Ask a Man: Arlene Dahl's Key to Femininity* (London: Frederick Muller Ltd, USA Prentice-Hall Inc, 1965), p.8

p.24 The Small, Private World of Audrey Hepburn in *Photoplay*, (February, 1957)

p.22 Sophia Loren in brainyquote.com/quotes/authors/s/sophia_loren.html

p.25 Audrey Hepburn in Pamela Keogh, *What Would Audrey Do?* (New York: Gotham Books 2008), p.105

p.25 Jeannette Wells, 'Did Designer Blast Nicole Kidman's Figure?' February 3, 2005, msnbc.msn.com

p.25 Nicole Kidman in Louise Burke, 'Nicole Kidman's Millionaire Boyfriends', *Sunday Mirror* (December 5, 2004)

p.25 Nicole Kidman on *The David Letterman Show*, (February 8, 2001)

p.28 Lou Schreiber in Julie Burchill, *Girls on Film* (London: Virgin Books, 1986), p.97

p.28 Sophia Loren in *Metro*, Monday (January 1, 2007)

p.28 Elizabeth Hurley in Natasha Walter, 'Lip-gloss and steel' *The Independent* (May 27, 2000)

p.28 Marilyn Monroe in Peter Noble and Yvonne Saxon, *Glamour: Film, Fashion and Beauty* (London: Burke, 1953), p.5

p.30 Elsie Pierce, *Be Beautiful: Hollywood Beauty Secrets* (Wisconsin: Whitman Publishing Co., 1933), p.5

p.32 Elizabeth Hurley in Polly Vernon, 'Gosh, I've got quite a lot of clothes on today.' *The Observer* (January 15, 2006)

p.32 Dolly Parton in Gordon Smart, 'Parton's Shock and Pwhoar.' *The Sun* (February 11, 2008)

p.33 Elizabeth Hurley in thinkexist.com/quotes/elizabeth_hurley/

p.34 Natalie Portman in uk.askmen.com/celebs/women/actress_60/64_natalie_portman.html

p.35 Elinor Glyn in Vincent L. Barnett, 'The novelist as Hollywood star: Author royalties and studio income in the 1920s.' *Film History: An International Journal* (Volume 20, Number 3, 2008), pp. 281–293)

p.40 Greta Garbo in garboforever.com/Garbo_Stories-33.htm

p.40 Spencer Tracy in *Pat and Mike* (1952) dir: George Cukor

p.40 Zadie Smith. 'The Divine Ms H' in *The Guardian* (July 1, 2003)

p.40 Madonna in Simon Doonan, 'Force of Nature.' *Elle* (May 2008)

p.42 Charlotte Church in brainyquote.com/quotes/authors/c/charlotte_church.html

p.43 Mae West in 'How Not to Wear a Tub'. *Time* (March 16, 1959)

p.43 Unknown critic in Jane Billinghurst, *Temptress : From the Original Bad Girls to Women on Top* (New York: Greystone Books, 2003), pp.159–60

p.44 Sophia Loren, *Women and Beauty* (London: Aurum Press, 1984), p.116

p.47 Ibid., p.121

p.47 Madonna interviewed on *Larry King Live* (October 10, 2002)

p.47 Catherine Zeta-Jones in howcelebritiesloseweight.com/catherine-zeta-jones-diet-and-exercise/

p.47 Charlize Theron in howcelebritiesloseweight.com/charlize-theron-diet-and-exercise/

p.47 Audrey Hepburn in Pamela Keogh, *What Would Audrey Do?* (New York: Gotham Books, 2008), p.106

p.48 Elizabeth Taylor in Peter Noble and Yvonne Saxon, *Glamour: Film, Fashion and Beauty* (London: Burke, 1953), p.7

p.48 Beyoncé Knowles in *New Zealand Herald* (November 18, 2008)

p.48 Shilpa Shetty in Julie McCaffrey and Fiona Cummins, 'Shilpa: My Style Secrets'. *Daily Mirror* (February 1, 2007)

p.48 Tyra Banks in 'I'm not a Size 2, so what?' *Shape* (June, 2007)

p.48 Twiggy in *The Times* (February 28, 2004)

p.49 Paige Thomas, *Beauty and Fashion* (Hollywood: Trend Books, 1957), p.105

p.53 Coco Chanel in Ross Care, The Little Black Dress' in Sara Pendergast (Editor) Tom Pendergast (Editor), *St. James Encyclopedia of Popular Culture* (Thomson Gale, 2002)

p.54 Audrey Hepburn in en.wikiquote.org/wiki/Audrey_Hepburn

p.57 Maurice Zolotow. *Marilyn: An Uncensored Biography* (London: W.H Allen, 1960), p.145

p.57 Joan Crawford in Louella Parsons. *L.A Examiner* (March, 1953)

p.59 Victoria Beckham in saidwhat.co.uk/keywordquotes/dress

p.60 Michael Kors in Merle Ginsberg, 'Dame Elizabeth Taylor and Michael Kors Talk Fashion.' *Harper's Bazaar* (August, 2006)

p.61 Kylie Minogue, Interview at Buckingham Palace, *The Royal Channel* (July 4, 2008)

p.62 Julie Burchill, *Diana* (London: Weidenfeld and Nicholson, 1998), p.62

p.65 Katharine Hepburn in William J. Mann, *Kate: The Woman Who Was Katharine Hepburn* (London: Faber & Faber, 2006), p.199

p.66 Mae West in Andrea Savardy, *Leading Ladies* (San Francisco: Chronicle Books, 2006), p.203

p.66 Dianne Brill. Boys, Boobs and High Heels: How to Get Dressed in Under Six Hours (London: Vermillion, 1992), p.54

p.67 Diane Brill. *Boys, Boobs and High Heels: How to Get Dressed in Under Six Hours* (London: Vermillion, 1992), p.60

p.67 Mae West in goodreads.com/quotes/show/68380

p.68 Edith Head in Paige Thomas, *Beauty and Fashion* (Hollywood: Trend Books, 1957), p.58

p.70 Gwen Stefani in prom.net/shoes

p.71 Marilyn Monroe in 'Something For the Boys' *Time* (August 11, 1952)

p.72 Bette Davis in Charlotte Chandler, *Bette Davis: The Girl Who Walked Alone* (London: Simon & Schuster, 2007), p.78

p.72 Reese Witherspoon in Hilary de Vries, 'Reese Witherspoon, What You Don't Know About Her' *Marie Claire* (September, 2005)

p.74 Joan Crawford, *My Way of Life* (New York: Simon & Schuster, 1971), p.57

p.75 Joan Crawford in Peter Hay, *Movie Anecdotes* (Oxford University Press, 1990), p.65

p.79 Arlene Dahl, *Always Ask a Man: Arlene Dahl's Key to Femininity* (London: Frederick Muller Ltd, USA Prentice-Hall Inc, 1965), pp.12–13

p.80 Dame Barbara Cartland, *The Pan Book of Charm* (London: Pan Books, 1965), p.5

p.81 Halle Berry in youtube.com/watch?v=NxLa73N6Rls

p.82 Dame Barbara Cartland, *The Pan Book of Charm* (London: Pan Books, 1965), p.88

p.82 Dolores del Rio in Patty Fox, *Star Style* (Santa Monica: Angel City Press, 1999), p.41

p.83 Bette Davis in 'Joan Crawford's Rollercoaster Life', *BBC News* (March 23, 2004)

p.85 Cecil Beaton in *US Vogue* (November, 1954)

p.85 Jane Fonda, *My Life So Far* (New York: Random House, 2006), p.557

p.87 John Robert Powers, *Secrets of Poise, Personality and Model Beauty* (New York: Prentice-Hall Inc, 1961), pp.234–7

p.91 Carla Bruni in Michael Roberts, Paris Match, *Vanity Fair* (September, 2008), p.172

p.92 Carla Bruni in John Hind, 'Did I say that? Carla Bruni-Sarkozy.' *The Observer on Sunday* (June 15, 2008)

p.92 Ibid.

p.95 Ronald Reagan in Jeanine Basinger, *The Star Machine* (New York: Alfred A. Knopf, 2007), p.314

p.95 Elizabeth Taylor in J. Randy Taraborrelli, *Elizabeth* (London: Pan Books, 2006), p.177

p.96 Ibid., p.396

p.96 Angelina Jolie in brainyquote.com/quotes/quotes/a/angelinajo167244.html

p.98 Jennifer Aniston in anistoncenter.com/jen/quotes/jennifer_on_others.php

p.98 Katharine Hepburn in William J. Mann, *Kate: The Woman Who Was Hepburn* (New York: Faber & Faber, 2006), p.155

p.98 James Brown in 'Davinia Taylor: Secrets of the Primrose Hill Set.' *Sunday Times* (June 8, 2008)

p.99 Davinia Taylor in 'Davinia Taylor: Secrets of the Primrose Hill Set.' *Sunday Times* (June 8, 2008)

p.99 Marlene Dietrich in Dr Scott Elliott, 'Character, commitment, compassion', *The Meridian Star* (February 21, 2009)

p.99 Dorothy Parker in answers.yahoo.com/question/index?qid=20081010132304AAxOGEf

p.99 Euripides in famousquotesandauthors.com/authors/euripides_quotes.html

p.99 Elizabeth Taylor in brainyquote.com/quotes/authors/e/elizabeth_taylor_2.html

p.99 Cher in brainyquote.com/quotes/authors/c/cher.html

p.99 Gwyneth Paltrow in scrapbook.com/quotes/doc/3402/258.html

p.100 Victoria Beckham in 'I Look Like a Miserable Cow.' *The Daily Mirror* (May 15, 2008)

p.101 John Robert Powers, *Secrets of Poise, Personality and Model Beauty* (New York: Prentice-Hall Inc, 1961), pp.8–9

p.106 Harry Meret in Paige Thomas, *Beauty and Fashion* (Hollywood: Trend Books, 1957), p.19

p.107 Marilyn Monroe in Peter Noble and Yvonne Saxon, *Glamour: Film, Fashion and Beauty* (London: Burke, 1953), p.5

p.114 Bette Davis in Charlotte Chandler, *Bette Davis: The Girl Who Walked Alone* (London: Simon & Schuster, 2007), p.14

p.115 Cecil Beaton and John Betjeman describing Joan Crawford's lips in Rosemarie Jarski, *Hollywood Wit* (London: Prion Books, 2000), p.149

p.118 Bette Davis in Charlotte Chandler, *Bette Davis: The Girl Who Walked Alone* (London: Simon & Schuster, 2007), p.78

p.118 Juliette Binoche in celebritybeautybuzz.com/index.php/2008/09/juliette-binoche-share

p.119 Charlotte Chandler, *Bette Davis: The Girl Who Walked Alone* (London: Simon & Schuster, 2007), p.12

p.120 Jean Kent, *Skin Deep: My Book of Beauty* (London: John Gifford Ltd, 1946), p.1

p.120 Marilyn Monroe, 'My Beauty Secrets' in *Photoplay* (October, 1953)

p.121 Cecil Beaton, *Cecil Beaton's Scrapbook 1937* (London: B.T Batsford), p.120

p.121 Brigitte Bardot in Tony Crawley, *Bebe: The Films of Brigitte Bardot* (London: Book Club Associates, 1977), p.40

p.121 Rosalind Russell in Paige Thomas, *Beauty and Fashion* (Hollywood: Trend Books, 1957), p.36

p.124 Cecil Beaton in Rosemarie Jarski, *Hollywood Wit* (London: Prion Books, 2000), p.149

p.124 Bette Davis in Charlotte Chandler, *Bette Davis: The Girl Who Walked Alone* (London: Simon & Schuster, 2007), p.78

p.125 'Barbara Stanwyck's Ear' in *Photoplay* (April, 1935)

p.126 Jean Kent, *Skin Deep: My Book of Beauty* (London: John Gifford Ltd, 1946), pp19–20

p.128 Marilyn Monroe, 'My Beauty Secrets' in *Photoplay* (October, 1953)

p.131 Bette Davis in Elsie Pierce, *Be Beautiful: Hollywood Beauty Secrets* (Wisconsin: Whitman Publishing Co., 1933), p.17

p.131 Angelina Jolie in *People* (May 11, 1998)

p.131 Monroe in in Peter Noble and Yvonne Saxon, *Glamour: Film, Fashion and Beauty* (London: Burke, 1953), p.5

p.131 Jean Kent, *Skin Deep: My Book of Beauty* (London: John Gifford Ltd, 1946), p.80

p.131 Elle Macpherson in Edwina Ings-Chambers, 'Elle Macpherson.' *The Financial Times* (December 2, 2006)

p.135 Joan Crawford in brainyquote.com/quotes/authors/j/joan_crawford.html

p.135 Jennifer Lopez in Bridget March, 'J.Lo: Posh's chop knocked me out.' *Cosmopolitan* (October, 2008)

p.136 Vidal Sassoon in *I'm Sorry I Kept You Waiting Madam* (London: Cassell, 1968), p.9

p137 Joan Crawford in Shaun Considine, *Bette and Joan: The Divine Feud* (New York, Dell Publishing, 1989), p.248

p.140 Jean Cocteau in 'Jean Cocteau on Bardot.' *Stop* (October, 1962)

p.142 Arlene Dahl, *Always Ask a Man: Arlene Dahl's Key to Femininity* (London: Frederick Muller Ltd, USA Prentice-Hall Inc, 1965), p.127

p.144 Parker Tyler, 'The Awful Fate of the Sex Goddess' in *Sex Psyche Etc in the Film* (London: Pelican, 1971), p.25

p.145 Ron Levine in *The Independent on Sunday* (27 June, 1999)

p.146 Gwen Stefani in 'Celebrity Central: Gwen Stefani.' *People* (March 12, 2009)

p.149 Sharon Osbourne on *Chelsea Lately* (October 11, 2008)

p.150 Arlene Dahl, *Always Ask a Man: Arlene Dahl's Key to Femininity* (London: Frederick Muller Ltd, USA Prentice-Hall Inc, 1965), p.127

p.151 Jean Kent, *Skin Deep: My Book of Beauty* (London: John Gifford Ltd, 1946), p.55

p.153 Greer Garson in Arlene Dahl, *Always Ask a Man: Arlene Dahl's Key to Femininity* (London: Frederick Muller Ltd, USA Prentice-Hall Inc, 1965), p.82

p.155 James Brown in forums.vogue.com.au/archive/index.php/t-142604.html

p.158 Joan Crawford in Elsie Pierce, *Be Beautiful: Hollywood Beauty Secrets* (Wisconsin: Whitman Publishing Co., 1933), p.8

p.158 Doris Day in Peter Noble and Yvonne Saxon, *Glamour:*

Film, Fashion and Beauty (London: Burke, 1953), p.20

p.160 Sarah Jessica-Parker in Julie Bindel, 'Things I've never done before: My first high heels' *The Guardian* (March 8, 2008)

p.161 Marilyn Monroe in Maurice Zolotow, *Marilyn Monroe: An Uncensored Biography* (London: W.H Allen & Co., 1960), p.127

p.161 Jimmy Starr in Anthony Summers, *Goddess: The Secret Lives of Marilyn Monroe* (London: Victor Gollancz Ltd, 1985), p.44

p.163 Jean Kent, *Skin Deep: My Book of Beauty* (London: John Gifford Ltd, 1946), p.3

p.164 Audrey Hepburn, 'The Small, Private World of Audrey Hepburn' *Photoplay* (February, 1957)

p.173 Elizabeth Taylor, *My Love Affair with Jewelry* (New York: Simon & Schuster, 2003)

p.175 Doris Day in Peter Noble and Yvonne Saxon, *Glamour: Film, Fashion and Beauty* (London: Burke, 1953), p.20

p.175 Ibid., p.33

p.181 Coco Chanel in Sameer Reddy, 'The Vulgar Game' *Newsweek* (January 10, 2009)

p.184 Constance Moore, *The Way to Beauty* (London: Ward Lock, 1955), p.31

p.191 La Belle Otero in Michael Harrison, *A Fanfare of Strumpets* (London: W.H Allen, 1971), p.187

p194 Mae West's screenplay for *Every Day's a Holiday* (1937)

p.202 Jean Cocteau, in Robert Andrews, *The Routledge Dictionary of Quotations* (London: Routledge, 1987), p.74

p.205 Diane Brill. *Boys, Boobs and High Heels: How to Get Dressed in Under Six Hours* (London: Vermillion, 1992), pp.10–11

p.206 Monroe in in Peter Noble and Yvonne Saxon, *Glamour: Film, Fashion and Beauty* (London: Burke, 1953), p.5

p.208 Lauren Bacall, *By Myself* (London: Jonathan Cape, 1979), p.94

p.208 Tallulah Bankhead, in Paul Taylor, 'THEATRE Tallulah!' in *The Independent* (July 4,1997)

p.208 Sharon Stone in Darryl Smith, 'No Dumb Blonde' in *The Sunday Post* (March 26, 2006)

p.210 Kylie Minogue in *B Magazine* (December, 2001)

p.210 Halle Berry acceptance speech in 'Halle Berry is the Sexiest Woman Alive' 2008. *Esquire* (October, 2008)

p.210 Drew Barrymore in interview with Julie Chen, CBS News (February 2, 2009)

p.210 Babe Paley on Pamela Harriman in Cynthia Robins, 'Mistresses and Muses', *San Francisco Chronicle* (June 30, 2001)

p.212 Monroe in in Peter Noble and Yvonne Saxon, *Glamour: Film, Fashion and Beauty* (London: Burke, 1953), p.5

p.213 Corinne Calvet in Peter Noble and Yvonne Saxon, *Glamour: Film, Fashion and Beauty* (London: Burke, 1953), p.18

p.214 Elle Macpherson in Edwina Ings-Chambers, 'FT Beauty: Elle Macpherson.' *The Financial Times* (December 2, 2006)

p.215 Jean Kent, *Skin Deep: My Book of Beauty* (London: John Gifford Ltd, 1946), p.24

p.218 Elle Macpherson in ellemacpherson.org/elle-macpherson-quotes.php

p.218 Sandra Bullock in *InStyle* (February, 2007)

p.220 Halle Berry in cinecon.com/news.php?id=0605251

p.220 Monroe in in Peter Noble and Yvonne Saxon, *Glamour: Film, Fashion and Beauty* (London: Burke, 1953), p.5

p.223 Irving Schulman, *Harlow: An Intimate Biography* (London: Mayflower, 1964), p.91

p.223 Judy Holliday in Lee Israel, 'Judy Holliday and the Red-Baiters: An Untold Story' in *Ms Magazine* (December, 1976)

p.224 Kathleen Hughes in Peter Noble and Yvonne Saxon,

Glamour: Film, Fashion and Beauty (London: Burke, 1953), p.61

p.226 Anon in Cornelia Otis Skinner, *Elegant Wits and Grandes Horizontals* (Cambridge: The Riverside Press, 1962), p.64

p.230 Juliette Binoche in Andrew Billen, 'True romantic is not so blue; Life is sweet for Juliette Binoche.' *The Sunday Herald* (March 4, 2001)

p.230 Katharine Hepburn in wisdomquotes.com/000985.html

p.231 Zsa Zsa Gabor in John Robert Colombo, *Columbo's Hollywood* (Toronto: Collins, 1979), p.106

p.234 Marilyn Monroe in *Pageant* (September, 1952)

p.235 Farley Granger in Peter Noble and Yvonne Saxon, *Glamour: Film, Fashion and Beauty* (London: Burke, 1953), p.70

p.238 Spike Milligan in Rosemarie Jarski, *Hollywood Wit* (London: Prion Books, 2000), p.172

p.238 Kitty Kelly, *Elizabeth Taylor: The Last Star* (New York: Simon & Schuster, 1981), p.195

p.241 Michelle Obama in Scott Fornek, 'He swept me off my feet' in *The Sun-Times* (October 3, 2007)

p.242 Christine Aguilera on *The Early Show*, CBS News (February 8, 2007)

p.242 Catherine Zeta-Jones in fhm.com/girls/covergirls/catherine-zeta-jones

p.242 Jerry Hall in Cosmo Landesman, 'Cosmo Landesman meets Jerry Hall.' *The Sunday Times* (November 21, 2004)

p.243 Paul Newman in Danny Miller, 'Remembering Paul Newman's Early Career.' *The Huffington Post* (September 29, 2008)

p.243 Simone Signoret in Florence Montreynaud, *Love: A Century of Love and Passion* (Cologne: Taschen, 1998), pp.239-40

p.244 Elizabeth Taylor in hellomagazine.com/profiles/elizabethtaylor/; The Ultimate Hollywood Trivia Guide in *Daily Mail* (26 December, 2007); in 'Serial Bride' in *The New York Times* (March 27, 2009) in brainyquote.com/quotes/authors/e/elizabeth_taylor.html; and in 'Our Eyes Have Fingers' in *Time* (December 25, 1964)

p.246 Tallulah Bankhead in Rosemarie Jarski, *Hollywood Wit* (London: Prion Books, 2000), p.142

p.246 Karl Lagerfeld in *Vanity Fair* (September 2008)

p.246 Carla Bruni in Kira Cochrane, 'Carla: How Britain fell for the French First Lady' in *The Guardian* (March 28, 2008)

p.246 Scarlett Johansson in *The People* (August 10, 2008)

p.247 Hedy Lamarr in hedy-lamarr.org/quotes.htm

p.247 Katharine Hepburn in Sheridan Morley, *Katherine Hepburn: A Celebration* (London: Pavilion, 1984), p.109

p.247 Beyoncé Knowles in beyonceknowles.org/quotes.php

p.248 Zsa Zsa Gabor in Matthew Sweet, 'The curious world of the first husband's club' in *The Independent* (19 February, 2002), p.248

p248 Bette Davis in Gary Herman, *The Book of Hollywood Quotes* (London: Omnibus Press, 1979), p.104

p.248 Reese Witherspoon in brainyquote.com/quotes/authors/r/reese_witherspoon.html

p.249 Jean Kent, *Skin Deep: My Book of Beauty* (London: John Gifford Ltd, 1946), p.27

Index

Page numbers in italic refer to the illustrations

A great many thanks to Dennis Norden for the generous use of his time and extensive library, Dianne Brill for her wit and glamour, Ian and Iona McCorquodale for the kind permission to use Dame Barbara Cartland's wise words, all at the London College of Fashion, my fabulous friends at Vidal Sassoon especially Josh Gibson, adorable literary agent Sheila Ableman, and, of course, at Quadrille, astute and very stylish Editorial Director Anne Furniss, Designer Claire Peters and Editor Katey Mackenzie.

Alicia M. Schweiger, Faiza Cochrane and Ilona Marten-McLean at Dianne Brill Cosmetics.

Editorial director Anne Furniss
Creative director Helen Lewis
Editor Katey Mackenzie
Designer Claire Peters
Illustrator Claire Peters
Picture assistant Samantha Rolfe
Production director Vincent Smith
Production controller Ruth Deary

First published in 2009 by
Quadrille Publishing Ltd
Alhambra House
27–31 Charing Cross Road
London WC2H 0LS
www.quadrille.co.uk

Reprinted in 2009, 2010
10 9 8 7 6 5 4 3

Text © 2009 Caroline Cox
Artwork, design and layout © 2009 Quadrille Publishing Ltd

British Library Cataloguing-in-Publication Data
A catalogue record for this book is available from the British Library.

ISBN: 978 184400 739 4

Printed in China

PICTURE CREDITS 2 Michael Ochs Archives/Getty Images; 8-9 Stockxpert; 17 © Sunset Boulevard/Corbis; 18 United Artists/ Courtesy of Getty Images; 20-21Stockxpert; 23 © DavisSeymour/ Magnum Photos; 37 Eugene Robert Richee/Getty Images; 38 Frazer Harrison/Getty Images; 45 Alfred Eisenstaedt/Time & Life Pictures/ Getty Images; 50-1Stockxpert; 55 Ezra Shaw/Getty Images; 56 M. Garrett/Murray Garrett/Getty Images; 64 © Bettmann/CORBIS; 73 © Mario Anzuoni/Reuters/Corbis; 76-7 Stockxpert; 84 © Bettmann/CORBIS; 93 Pool/Anwar Hussein Collection/Wireimage; 94 Theo Kingma/Rex Features; 102-3 Stockxpert; 111© Bettmann/ CORBIS; 112 © Mario Anzuoni/Reuters/Corbis; 129 Dave Hogan/ Getty Images; 130 Carlos Alvarez/Getty Images; 132-3 Stockxpert; 141 Keystone/Getty Images; 147 © Stephane Cardinale/People Avenue/Corbis; 148 Fred Duval/FilmMagic; 156-7 Stockxpert; 165 Hulton Archive/Getty Images; 168 Bill Davila/Rex Features; 176 SNAP/Rex Features; 178-9 Stockxpert; 185 © CORBIS; 186 Alfred Eisenstaedt/Time & Life Pictures/Getty Images; 197 Michael Ochs Archives/Getty Images; 200-1 Stockxpert; 203 © Stephane Cardinale/People Avenue/Corbis; 209 © Bettmann/CORBIS; 221 c.U.A./Everett/Rex Features; 222 Margaret Chute/Getty Images; 228-9 Stockxpert; 239 © Bettmann/CORBIS; 240 TIMOTHY A. CLARY/AFP/Getty Images; 254 SNAP/Rex Features